Broodmare Reproduction

for the Equine Practitioner

William B. Ley, DVM, MS, DACT

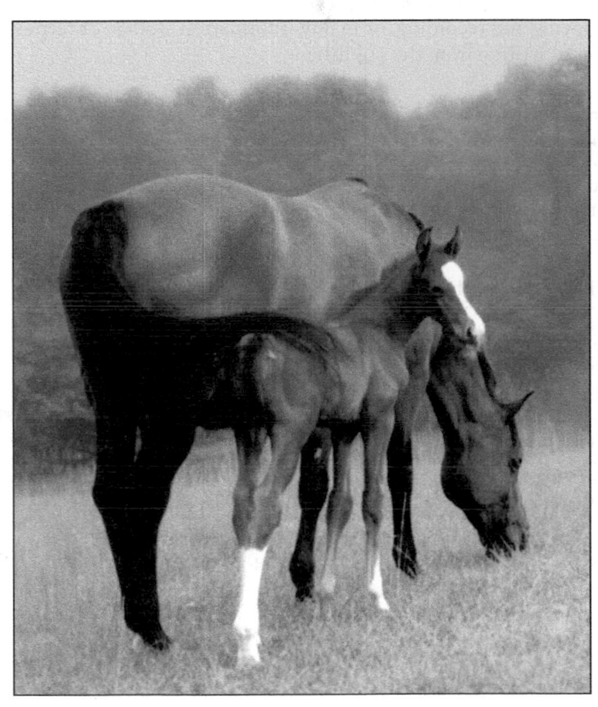

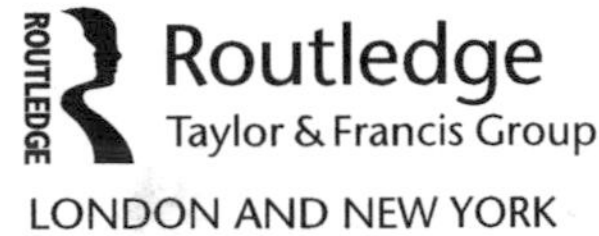

LONDON AND NEW YORK

Executive Editor: Carroll C. Cann
Development Editor: Susan L. Hunsberger
Editor: Cynthia Roantree
Creative Director: Anita B. Sykes
Illustrator and Diagnostic Photos: Gail D. Maslyk, www.equinegraphics.com
Production & Layout: 5640 Design, www.fiftysixforty.com

First published 2004 by Teton NewMedia

Published 2019 by Routledge
2 Park Square, Milton Park, Abingdon, Oxon OX14 4RN
52 Vanderbilt Avenue, New York, NY 10017

Routledge is an imprint of the Taylor & Francis Group, an informa business

ISBN 978-1-59161-011-3 (pbk)

Library of Congress Cataloging-in-Publication Data

Ley, William B.
Broodmare reproduction for the equine practitioner/William B. Ley.
p. cm. -- (Made easy series)
Includes bibliographical references and index.
ISBN 1-591610-11-7
1. Horses-Reproduction. 2. Horses-Breeding. 3. Veterinary obstetrics. I. Title. II. Made easy series (Jackson, Wyo.)

SF768.2.H67L49 2003
636.1'08982--dc21

2003047382

Dedication

To my family, friends, mentors, associates, and clients who have helped and inspired me along this journey. Most important to my professional development, I would like to thank and acknowledge Drs. Jim Bowen, Jim Voss, Ed Squires, John Hughes, and Peter Chenoweth.

...and to the many horses who have helped me learn, Thank You!

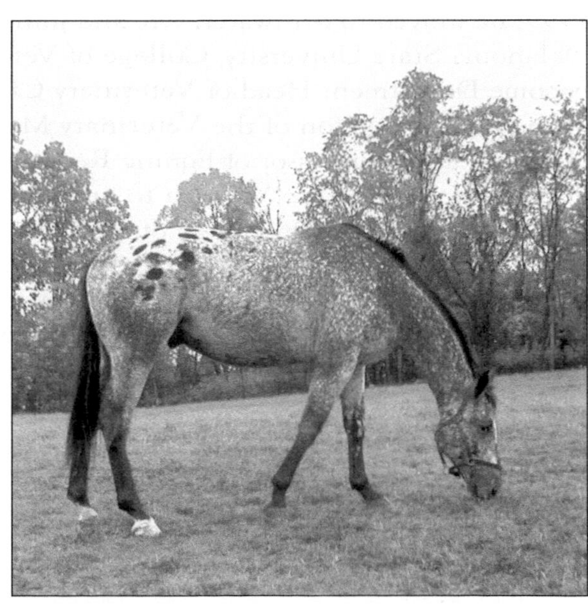

About the Author

Dr. Bill Ley is a graduate of Colorado State University College of Veterinary Medicine, where he received a bachelor's degree in Veterinary Science and then his doctoral degree (DVM) in 1978. He completed an internship in Equine Medicine and Reproduction at the University of California at Davis, CA (1978-1979). and residency program training in Large Animal Theriogenology (with emphasis in equine) at Texas A & M University, College Station, TX (1979-1981). During his residency, he received the Master of Science degree with his research and thesis on equine endometrial cytology. Following this, he spent two years in private equine practice in Iowa (Tri-State Veterinary Clinic, 1981-1983), and two breeding seasons as a Resident Veterinarian at Graham Farm's Southwest Stallion Station (1983-1984), standing Rocket Wrangler, Scott's Poppy, and Mr. Dark Jet. He joined the faculty at the Virginia-Maryland Regional College of Veterinary Medicine, Blacksburg, Virginia in 1984, where he was engaged in clinical teaching, equine research, and field service programs of the Veterinary Teaching Hospital in Equine Production Management Medicine (Equine Medicine and Reproduction). He became a Diplomate of the American College of Theriogenologists in 1985. In August of 1999, he moved to Stillwater, OK and joined the faculty at Oklahoma State University, College of Veterinary Medicine, to become Department Head of Veterinary Clinical Sciences, Head of the Equine Section of the Veterinary Medical Teaching Hospital, and a Professor of Equine Reproduction. In the summer of 2002, he returned to Virginia to enter private practice. He is now the veterinarian in charge of the Regional Equine Associates Central Hospital (REACH) in northern Virginia, an intermediate-care, emergency and referral clinic near Millwood, VA. He is establishing an equine-only reproductive specialty referral practice at the same location.

Further information can be obtained by visiting his web site at: http://www.horse-repro.com

Preface

Reproduction plays a prominent role in equine private practice. Breeding problems and their resolution are a frequent challenge to many practitioners. This book is intended to serve as a practical basis to aid students, new graduates, mixed animal practitioners, and equine emphasis veterinarians alike in their understanding and management of broodmares.

The book is not intended to be an all-inclusive reference text for equine reproductive problems. Rather the basics are presented as a foundation, a solid base, on which to build during your life-long learning process. I firmly believe that we do not know or understand all there is to know. We must confront the challenges of our profession with an open mind, a curiosity for new events and findings, a willingness to admit we do not have an answer to every question, and the dedication to seek an answer whenever and wherever possible.

I never cease to be amazed by the challenges and intricacies of life, especially in relation to its initiation at conception. But the challenges and wonderment do not stop there. Preserving and optimizing the quality of life of our equine companions has and will continue to be a life-long personal quest.

I extend to you the invitation to correspond with me concerning this text or any question you may have regarding broodmare reproduction. If I don't have an immediate answer, I promise to extend every reasonable effort in an attempt to assist you.

Bill Ley
DrLey@horse-repro.com

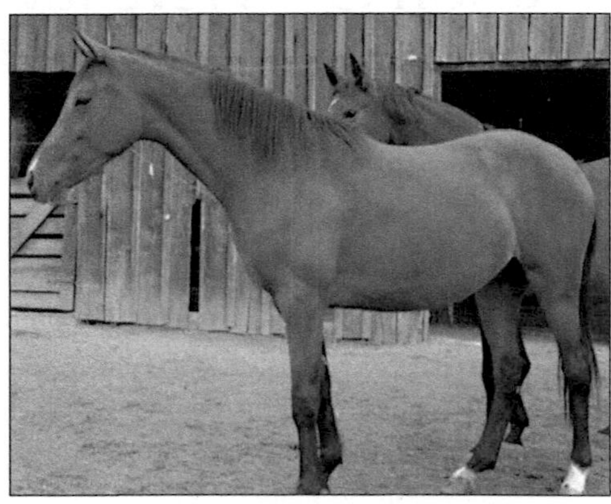

Table of Contents

Section 1 Equine Reproductive Efficiency

Section 2 Breeding Management Systems

Section 3 Preventive Medicine Program for Broodmares

Section 4 Anatomy and Physiology

Section 5 Seasonality, the Estrous Cycle and its Manipulation and Artificial Control

Section 6 Breeding Serviceability Exam of the Mare

Section 7 Breeding Management

Section 8 Pregnancy Diagnosis

Section 9 Early Embryonic Loss

Section 10 Infectious Causes of Endometritis and Treatment Options

Section 11 Non-infectious Causes of Infertility

Section 12 Assisted Reproductive Technologies

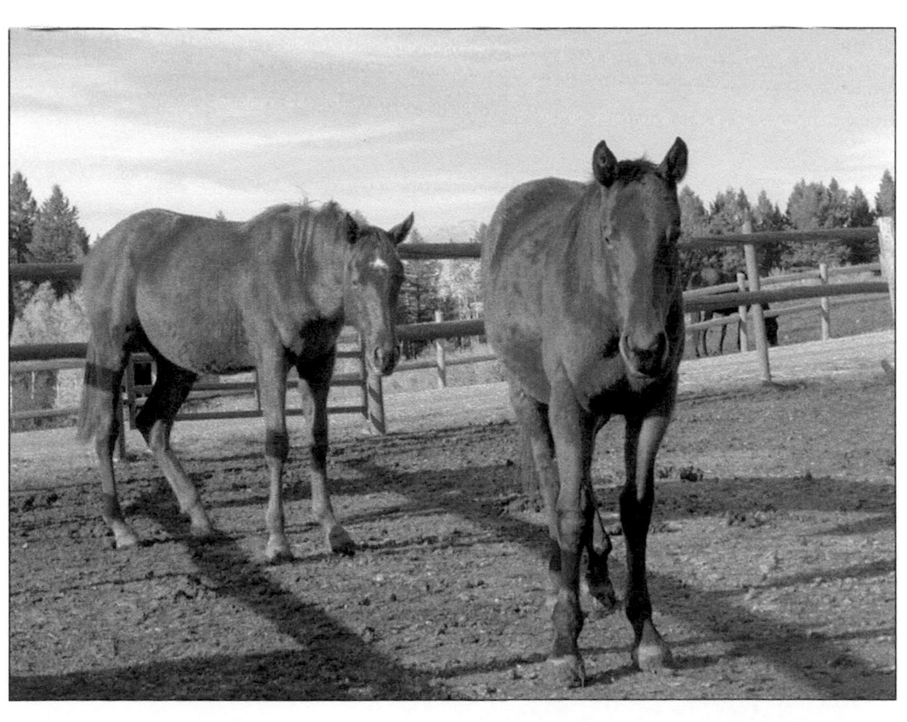

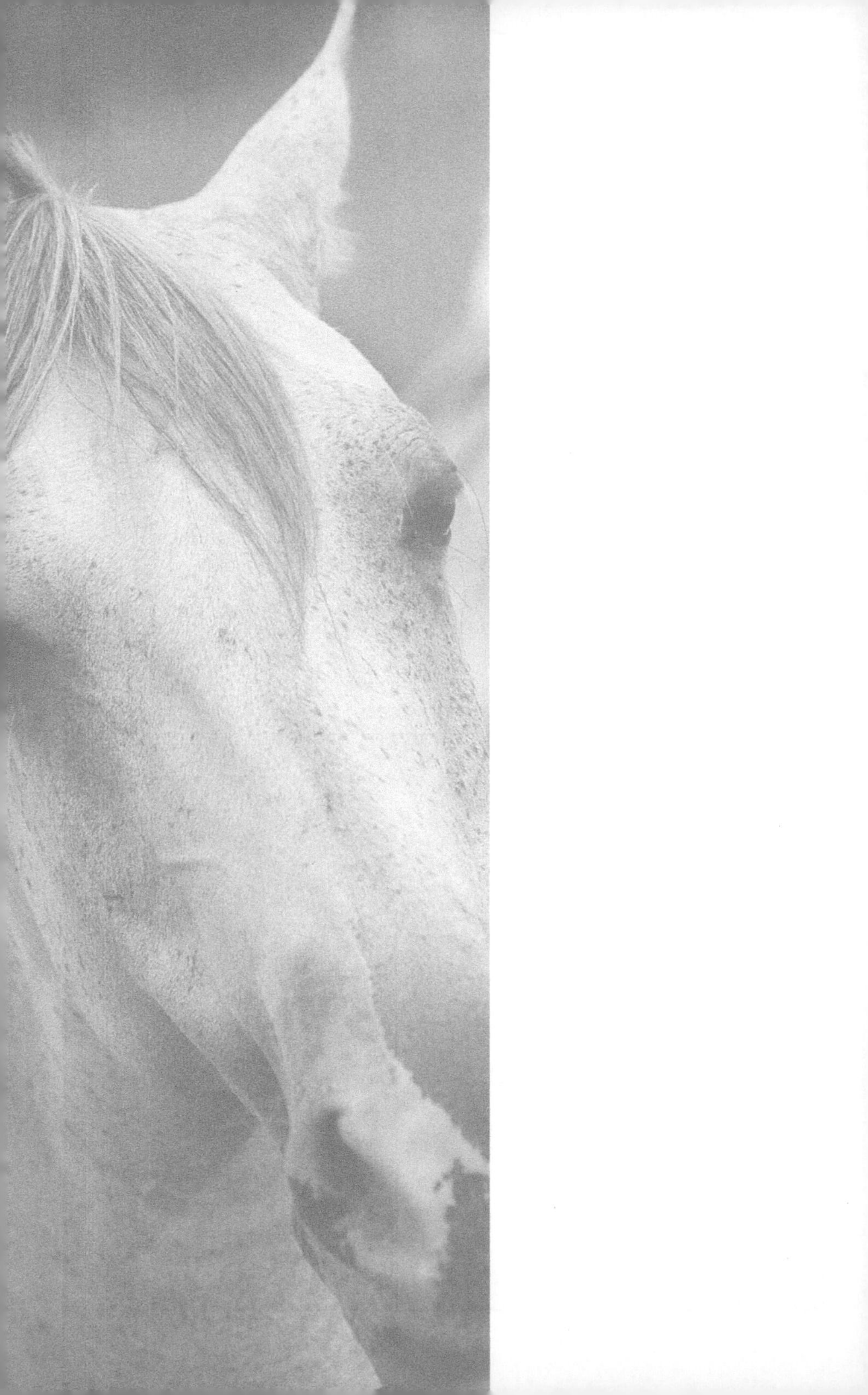

Section 1

Equine Reproductive Efficiency

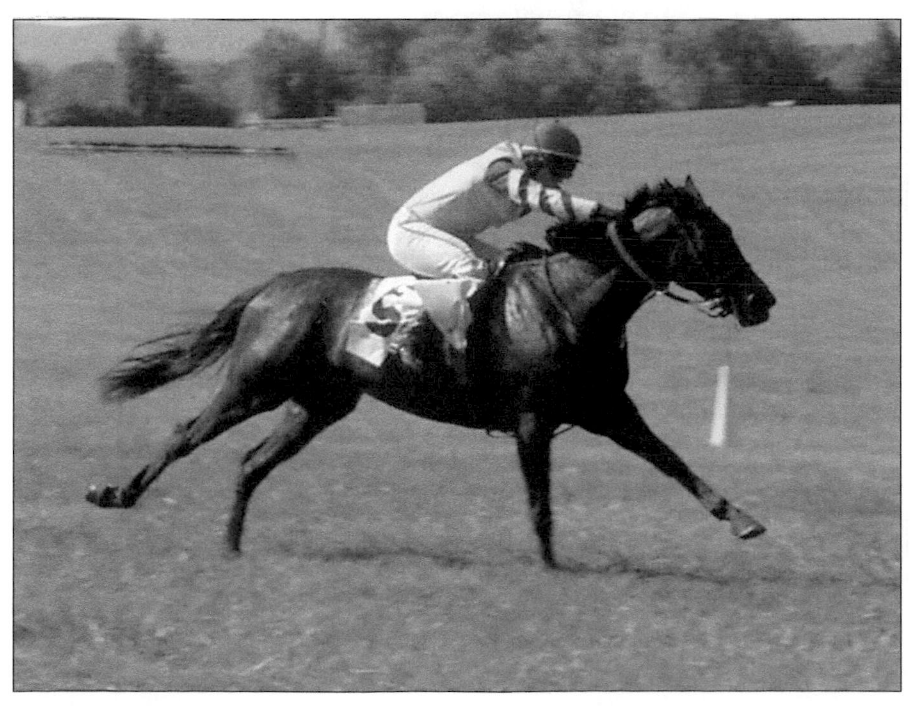

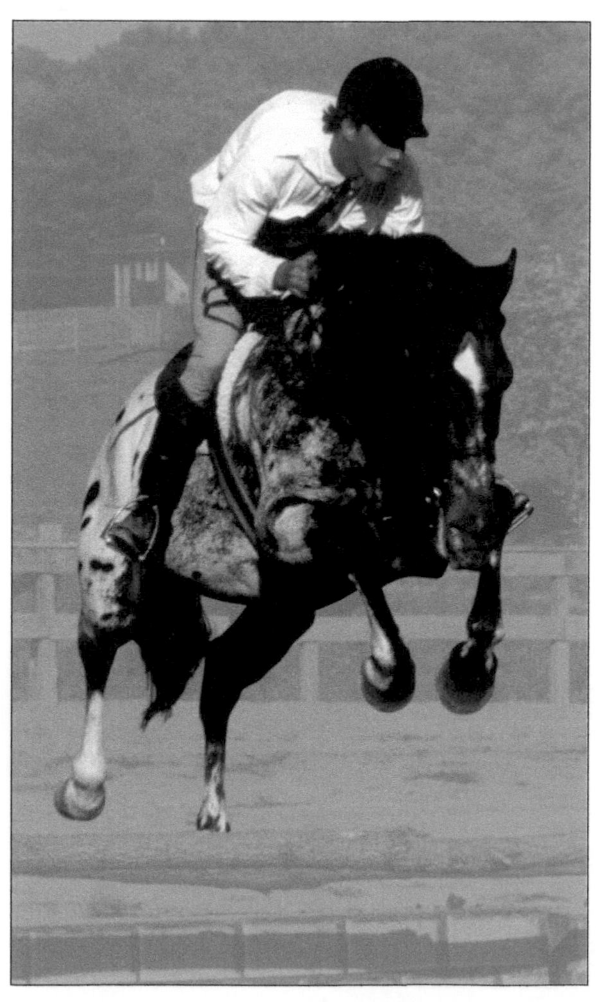

General Principles

The primary goal of this book is to provide a useful and concise reference on broodmare reproduction and breeding management for veterinarians and veterinary students. An attempt is made here to present key features and facts in a concise format, but the practice of veterinary medicine, and most especially equine reproduction, is also an art. Practicing an art and being competent, as well as successful, requires years of practical experience. Do not become discouraged in your attempts that may prove disheartening, learn from them. Remembering always that you are dealing with nature, and one of its more complex biological systems. Try as we might, recipes, formulas, definitions, rules, guidelines, expectations, and methods of therapy do not always work or apply in every circumstance or situation. Be creative, find the beauty in procreation, and always seek to learn.

Some Helpful Hints

Scattered throughout the text, you will find the following symbols to help you focus on what is routine and what may be really important:

✓ This is a routine feature or basic point for understanding the subject discussed.

🔑 The key symbol will be used selectively to indicate a very important point to assist your understanding of the topic area.

✋ Stop. This does not look important, but it can really make a difference when trying to sort out unusual or difficult situations. It can be my opinion based on personal experience.

💣 Something serious will happen if you do not remember this, possibly resulting in injury or loss to the patient, and upset to the client.

⊙ A companion CD is available for purchase by calling 877-306-9793. The CD contains the full text, figures, and tables of this book formatted for easy search and retrieval. The CD symbol indicates that additional images and video of a topic are available on the CD or a hyperlink reference for further reading.

Success in equine reproduction depends on a solid understanding of reproductive anatomy, physiology, endocrinology, breeding management, disease prevention and treatment as indicated, and the maintenance of complete and accurate records.

An understanding of optimal reproductive efficiency in the horse serves as a sound basis for communicating with clients the expected normal. Having this understanding makes the identification of abnormal performance much easier.

Definitions

✓ *Fertility:* the quality or state of being fertile, which means producing or being capable of producing offspring; it implies the power or ability to reproduce in kind or to assist in reproduction and growth.

A mare with appropriate anatomic, physiologic, and endocrine structure and function has the ability or implied power to reproduce. She by definition then would be considered fertile. But she may be terribly inefficient at the task given loss, damage, injury or disease to an integral anatomic structure, or a dysfunction in her underlying reproductive physiology. It is therefore preferable to avoid defining the mare's ability to reproduce as either fertile or infertile. A mare that has undergone bilateral ovariectomy can effectively be used as an embryo transfer recipient mare and therefore has retained the ability to reproduce in kind. She must by definition be considered fertile, yet has no inherent ability remaining to conceive on her own.

✓ *Efficiency:* the quality or degree of being efficient, which means productive of the desired effect, especially productive without waste.

🗝 *Reproductive efficiency:* the ability to produce offspring in a positive and effective manner without waste.

It would be agreed to by many that an 8 year old mare is likely to be more efficient at producing an offspring than a 24 year old mare. Both are, or have the likelihood of being, fertile. Many 24 year old mares produce live offspring, yet their efficiency at the task is considerably much less than that of the 8 year old mare. The younger mare typically requiring much fewer resources in terms of labor, time, pharmaceuticals, and breeding attempts to achieve conception and gestate her fetus to full term than the older mare.

✓ *Soundness* implies an 'absolute' understanding, which when used for the purpose of a mare's breeding soundness examination, is potentially misleading. Its use should be avoided in this context, as it is extremely difficult, if not impossible, to absolutely state from an examination that a mare without reservation can and will conceive and carry her fetus to full term. The likelihood may exist; there may be no findings to indicate any other probable outcome than success, but a likelihood and a probability are not absolute.

✓ *Suitable* is a 'term of art' and refers to temperament, ability, and relationship of the horse to rider, driver, exhibitor or other desired use. While a breeding suitability examination may be more useful terminology, it is not entirely appropriate for the veterinarian to pass judgement on suitability with respect to the mare's genetics for breeding purposes.

🗝 *Serviceable* is the most useful term as it implies the relationship of physical capability to intended use. It is the most appropriate term to use in the context of the veterinarian's performance of an examination, the opinion or recommendation of which relates to the present relationship of the mare's physical (and physiological) capability to be used as a reproductively efficient broodmare.

Reproductive efficiency and breeding serviceability in the mare therefore require the presence of normal and functional anatomic reproductive tract components with reasonable physiologic function. These performing as nature intended enable her to undergo regular estrous cycles, exhibit estrous behavior, ovulate a normally matured ovum (ova), and transport the ovulated ova to the site of fertilization. She must have the uterine environment to support or allow normal sperm transport at breeding time and sperm capacitation following semen deposition. The viable ovum in the appropriate environment and timing with viable capacitated spermatozoa then set up the opportunity for conception to occur. The mare's uterine environment must then have the ability to recover from the challenge of breeding or insemination in time to receive the conceptus or embryo 6-8 days after fertilization. The mare must recognize that she is indeed pregnant, and sustain in utero embryonic and fetal growth, cooperate effectively with placental growth, function and development, and have the anatomic ability to produce a viable offspring by spontaneous unassisted vaginal delivery. She must further be capable of supporting her foal's extrauterine growth through lactation for a defined period of time until weaning. During the immediate postpartum time, and while lactating, she must also involute the uterus, cycle again, be receptive to breeding, and conceive again for the following year's production of offspring. How serviceable for such events and how efficiently she can perform them are dependent upon a multitude of factors. Factors which in a natural environment (e.g., pasture breeding) can come together making her wonderfully efficient. Under the influences of domestication, husbandry, and breeding management (e.g., breeding in hand) she can become very inefficient.

✓ *Maiden:* a mare that has never been bred or exposed to a stallion for breeding purposes. It usually implies a young mare, but many mid- to late-teenage mares used in performance may also fit into this definition. Young maiden mares having gone through puberty are typically the most reproductively efficient.

✓ *Lactating:* a mare that has 'proven' herself, has a foal at her side, and is lactating; the result of having recently conceived, successfully gestated, and foaled. She may also be referred to as a 'wet', foaling, or postpartum mare. They are most typically reproductively efficient, but advancing age or foaling injury may make them less likely to conceive and produce another offspring in the next 12 months.

✓ *Barren:* a mare that has failed to conceive in the most recent breeding season, or one more distant and not since. She may have conceived, been confirmed as pregnant, and then subsequently aborted, or had a stillbirth, and fit into the barren category. Key to this is having had the opportunity to conceive and carry to term, yet has failed to do so. They are therefore less reproductively efficient than the preceding two groups of mares.

Rates, Terms, and Efficiency

✓ The best measure of breeding performance is the live foal crop. This is defined as the proportion of the number of live healthy foals produced compared to the number of mares maintained for breeding in a given season or period of time. The most widely used basis (i.e., denominator) for calculating the live foal crop is the number of mares actually bred or having had the opportunity for exposure to a reproductively fit or efficient stallion (or his spermatozoa). On the basis of mares bred, the live foal crop should be 75-80%.

✓ The proportion of mares slated for breeding that are not actually bred during a given season should rarely exceed 5% (i.e., for medical reasons).

🗝 *Conception rate (CR)* is defined as the number of mares that are diagnosed pregnant between 9-17 days post-ovulation compared with the total number of mares bred. This parameter may be calculated based on a single estrous cycle, or monthly, or seasonal intervals.

✓ Conception rate can be influenced by techniques of breeding such as natural service (NS) versus artificial insemination (AI). These are further influenced by other factors such as number of natural covers or inseminations per estrus, use of routine veterinary reproductive examinations, reproductive status of each mare (e.g., lactating, barren, maiden), postpartum management of lactating mares, age of the individual mare, and individual stallion reproductive efficiency.

✓ Conception rate on a per estrous cycle basis refers to the proportion of mares that conceive when bred in a given estrous period. This can be calculated based on the first cycle of the season, the second cycle, cumulative for a month, or an entire season. This parameter includes only those mares bred at each individual estrous period and provides information on efficiency of conception.

✓ The average number of estrous periods bred per conception is 1.7.

✓ The number of covers per estrous period is a matter of management efficiency. Such factors as NS versus AI and the individual stallion's sperm longevity may come into play, but covers or services per estrous period usually should not exceed an average of 1.1.

✓ *Seasonal (or cumulative) conception rate* signifies the proportion of mares that conceive during the course of the breeding season compared to the number of mares bred or exposed to the stallion. The seasonal CR of mares can be expected to exceed 90%.

✓ Conception rates at first breeding will be the highest approaching 60-65%. At the second cycle a similar percentage of the remaining group of eligible nonpregnant mares can be expected to conceive. But by the third cycle, only 45-50% will conceive and will continue a downward trend from there until the sixth cycle where less than 10% actually conceive.

✓ Foaling (postpartum, wet, or lactating) mares may not follow this pattern. The fertility of postpartum mares improves markedly after the first postpartum estrous cycle (foal heat) and may continue to improve over the next 1 to 2 cycles. The average CR may not decrease markedly over several sequential postpartum estrous periods for this group of mares.

✓ Early conception is one of the most significant factors in sustaining high levels of broodmare reproductive efficiency year after year. A desirable distribution over the months of the typical breeding season would be as follows: Feb 35-40%; Mar 65-70%; Apr 80%; May 85%; June 75%.

✓ The average interval between sequential foalings per broodmare must be maintained at 12 months or less. When mares foal well into the breeding season, a period not greater than 20-30 days between foaling and diagnosis of conception is needed to maintain a 12-month foaling interval. The exception is when a mare foals in January. The distance from foaling to conception can be lengthened without penalizing the overall seasonal performance. Good reproductive performance is a short interval from foaling to conception coupled with a high seasonal CR and PR. Under good management, the interval from the first postpartum breeding to diagnosis of conception will range from 10-30 days.

✓ Gestation length may vary from mare to mare, breed to breed, time of the year that the mare is due to foal, and nutrition (e.g., fescue mycotoxicosis or poor nutrition may both prolong gestational length). Mares conceiving early in the season have longer gestational periods than those that conceive later in the season. Artificial lighting programs can reduce gestational length by as much as 10 days without harm to the foal's viability.

🗝 *Pregnancy rate (PR)* is defined as the number of mares pregnant at day 45 (or beyond) compared with the total number of mares bred. This parameter may be calculated based on single estrous cycle, monthly, or seasonal intervals.

It is important to note that many horsemen and even veterinarians use conception rate and pregnancy rate interchangeably, which often confuses interpretations of reproductive efficiency. It further confuses an investigation into decreased reproductive performance on a farm since the laxity in terminology and a lack of understanding of their true meaning can lead to false impressions. Just as accuracy in records keeping is integral to a successful breeding program, so is accuracy in terminology.

Factors Influencing Pregnancy Rate (PR)

✓ Length of estrus: Mares have a greater probability or risk of becoming pregnant when they have a longer estrus (e.g., 6 vs. 4 days in heat). There may not be a significant difference in PR between mares that are in estrus from 2 to 9 days, but PR will decline when estrus duration exceeds 9 days.

✓ Number of inseminations or covers: Mares that become pregnant are typically inseminated a greater number of times (3.3 vs. 2.8) per cycle than those that do not become pregnant. The opportunity for conception and therefore pregnancy is a "numbers game."

✓ Timing of insemination or cover: When all mares are considered, PR is better for those mares that are inseminated on the last day of estrus. The opportunity for conception and therefore pregnancy is "timing game."

✓ The stallion: The per cycle pregnancy rate for proven stallions ranges from 60 to 65%; the range for all stallions can vary from 0 to 75% (occasionally greater).

🗝 Factors having a significant positive influence on PR: Younger mares aged 6 to 10 years, a stallion breeding frequency of once 2 days prior to breeding the mare in question (the numbers game again).

🗝 Factors having a significant negative influence on PR: Mares aged 15 or older, the use of a post-breeding infusion, the use of semen extender, barren reproductive status, breeding dates after the beginning of May, positive or inflammatory uterine cytology result, positive uterine swab culture result, an individual stallion of low fertility.

✓ Pregnancy rates per season (cumulative) are usually greater than 90%; an acceptable range is from 80 to 100%.

✓ The range of estrous periods bred per live foal is between 2.0-2.5. The difference between this and the average number of estrous periods bred per conception (i.e., 1.7; see above) represents reproductive loss, the most important of which is early embryonic loss or early embryonic death.

🗝 Early embryonic death (EED): Defined as the loss of the conceptus or embryo between days 9 to 45, usually after day 18 and before day 36.

✓ Up to 20% of equine embryos present at day 11 may not survive to day 15. An additional 7-13% present at day 15 may be lost between days 15 and 45. One large study in Quarter Horse mares and stallions reported an 11.0 to 11.5 % EED rate.

✓ In lactating mares, early embryonic losses were associated with early conception after foaling and with the stage of lactation. This is especially true if mares were covered in their foal heat. This may reflect a competition between the nutritional demand of lactation and the growing embryo, losses due to incomplete uterine involution during the postpartum period, or subclinical endometritis undetected prior to breeding.

Causes of Early Embryonic Death (EED)

✓ Intrinsic factors: Endocrine, oviductal, uterine, maternal age, or barren reproductive status

✓ Extrinsic factors: Physiologic stress, nutrition, season, environmental stress, temperature, sire, or iatrogenic

✓ Embryonic factors: Twinning and chromosomal abnormality or defect

<u>Age of mare:</u> Reproductive efficiency increases in mares as they age from 2 to 7 years, plateau from 8 to 13 years of age, and decline thereafter through mid to late 20s. Aged mares (i.e., > 15) are less likely to produce a foal from each cycle bred, or even each season bred. It is advisable to minimize the number of covers or inseminations in these mares and to breed these mares to the most reproductively efficient stallions.

<u>Normal rates of pregnancy loss:</u> Losses greater than 5% after 45 days gestation and prior to term are cause for concern.

✓ <u>Causes of pregnancy loss:</u> Relative progesterone deficiency (or other endocrine abnormality), twin pregnancy, viral infections causing abortion (e.g., EHV-1/4, EAV), placentitis (e.g., viral, bacterial, fungal), gestational abnormalities (e.g. umbilical torsion, congenital defects, toxin-induced fetal damage, hydrallantois, hydramnios), difficulty at foaling (e.g., dystocia, stillbirth, fescue grass mycotoxicity).

✓ Early embryonic death loss in the mare will be further discussed in Section 9.

⊙ A sample of parameters to evaluate when making an evaluation of a farm's reproductive efficiency is provided in Table 1-1. This can be used in comparison to the various published reproductive efficiency rates summarized in Table 1-2. See CD for a list of additional recommended reading, some of which have hyperlinks to abstracts or full text articles.

Table 1-1
Example Parameters for Evaluation of Reproductive Efficiency

PARAMETER	FARM OVERALL	STALLIONS			
		A	B	C	D
Mares bred (No.)					
Mares bred (%)					
Cycles serviced (No.)					
Cycles serviced (%)					
Pregnancies (No.)					
Cycles/Pregnancy (%)					
Cumulative PR (%)					
Adjusted PR (%)[1]					
EED's* (No.)					
EED Rate (%)					
Adjusted EED Rate (%)[2]					
Twins (No.)					
Twin Rate (%)					
Mares bred at foal heat (No.)					
Mares bred at FH (%)					
Pregnant to FH breeding (No.)					
Cumulative PR at FH (%)					
EED's at FH Breeding (No.)					
EED rate at FH (%)					

*EED = early embryonic death loss
[1] Adjusted for EED losses
[2] Adjusted for losses at Foal Heat breeding

Table 1-2
Reproductive Efficiency Indices in the Horse

Single Service:

PARAMETER	BREED[1]	METHOD[2]	PERCENTAGE
CR[3]	QH	AI	74.1
PR[4]	QH	AI	51
PR	TB	NS	43

Cumulative/Seasonal:

PARAMETER	BREED	METHOD	PERCENTAGE
CR	StB	AI	83.1
CR	StB	NS	74.5
CR	QH	AI	82.5
CR	TB	NS	73.2

Cumulative/Seasonal:

PARAMETER	BREED	METHOD	NUMBER
Services/conception	StB	AI	1.5
Services/conception	StB	AI	1.6
Services/conception	QH	AI	1.4
Services/conception	TB	NS	2.6
Services/conception	TB	NS	3.2

PARAMETER	BREED	PERCENTAGE
EED	Multiple	13
EED	TB	8.4
EED	QH	3.1
EED	ASB	14.7
	Pregnancy Type	
EED	singleton	13
EED	twins	24

continued

Table 1-2 continued

First Service:

Parameter	Status	Breed	Percentage
PR	Maiden	QH	48
PR	Maiden	TB	38
PR	Barren	QH	46
PR	Barren	TB	34
PR	Lactating (all)	Unk	56
PR	Lactating (all)	TB	51
PR	Lactating at foal heat	QH	58
PR	Lactating at foal heat	TB	41
PR	Lactating not at foal heat	QH	65
PR	Lactating not at foal heat	TB	67

Cumulative/seasonal:

Parameter	Breed	Method	Percentage
PR	QH	NS	88.3
PR	TB	NS	75.2
PR	TB	NS	80.6
PR	TB	NS	65.1
PR	StB	NS	62.9
PR	App	NS	81.2
PR	Arab	NS	81.3
PR	Multiple	NS and AI	54

Parameter	Status	Breed	Percentage
PR	Maiden	QH	89
PR	Maiden	TB	76
PR	Maiden	Multiple	58
PR	Maiden	Multiple	78.6
PR	Barren	QH	82
PR	Barren	TB	66
PR	Barren	Multiple	47
PR	Barren	Multiple	72.4
PR	Lactating	QH	87
PR	Lactating	TB	80
PR	Lactating	Multiple	56
PR	Lactating	Multiple	79.5

continued

Table 1-2 continued

Cumulative/Seasonal:

Parameter	Breed	Method	Percentage
Foaling rate	StB	AI	73.8
Foaling rate	StB	NS	68.7
Foaling rate	StB	NS	59.5
Foaling rate	QH	NS	83.3
Foaling rate	TB	NS	66.3
Foaling rate	TB	NS	69.7
Foaling rate	TB	NS	58.2
Foaling rate	App	NS	90.1
Foaling rate	Arab	NS	79.5

From multiple references listed in Further Reading; each reference had a minimum of 100 mares included in the survey.

[1] Breed: QH: American Quarter Horse; TB: Thoroughbred; StB: Standardbred; Arab: Arabian, ASB: American Saddlebred; App: Appaloosa; Unk: Unknown.

[2] Method: NS: Natural service; AI: Artificial Insemination.

[3] Conception rate (CR) defined by rectal palpation (or ultrasonography when available) prior to day 30.

[4] Pregnancy rate (PR) defined by same method(s) as for CR, but at or after day 45.

Section 2
Breeding Management Systems

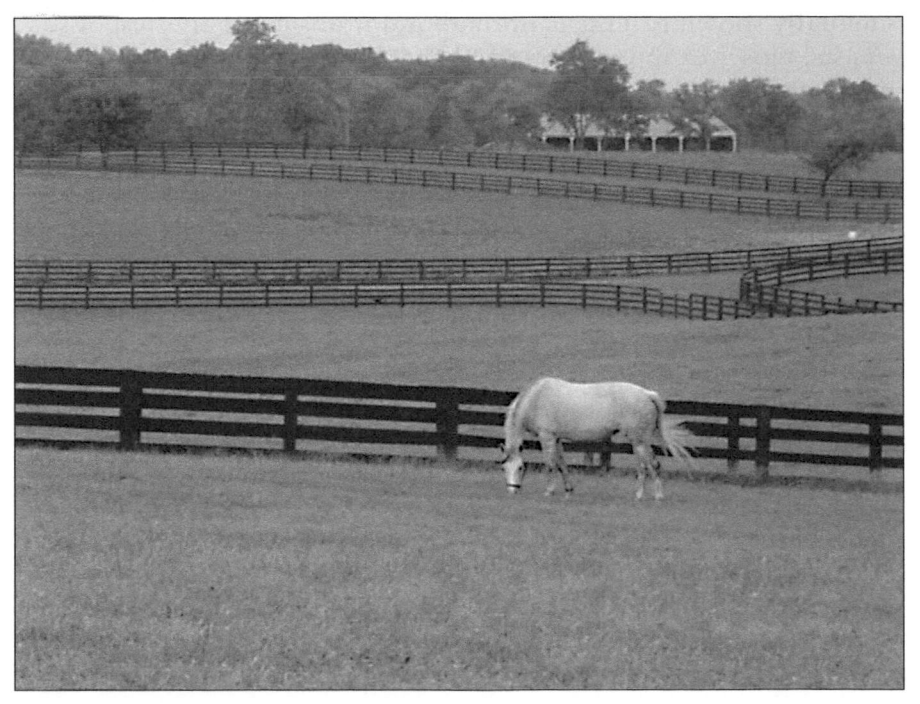

Successful breeding management for the mare requires a reliable system for estrous detection (i.e., teasing program), accuracy in determining ovulation time(s), a natural service or artificial insemination delivering an optimal number of viable sperm to the site of fertilization, good breeding hygiene to minimize reproductive disease transmission, optimal nutrition, and excellent records management.

Terms and Terminology

✓ Estrus: The physiologic period or condition dominated by a large follicle (or more than one follicle) that is approaching ovulation under the primary influence of estrogen; behaviorally the female is receptive to breeding. Also known as in heat, teasing in, hot, or showing.

🗝 Diestrus: The physiologic period or condition dominated by a corpus luteum (CL) under the primary influence of progesterone and behaviorally not receptive to breeding. Also known as cold, out, not showing, not in, or not in heat.

✓ Grey areas in behavioral signs of estrus or diestrus occur during the transition from one to the other which can last from 1 to 4 days resulting in questionable interpretation of what the mare is actually showing. This is normal and if unsure or the response persists, closer examination of the mare's internal reproductive tract is warranted. Also known as coming in, going out, unsure, or questionable.

✓ The mare is seasonally polyestrous, which means there is a defined period of time during the year in which she exhibits cyclical or repetitive signs of estrus in response to her reproductive physiology as determined by follicle development, production of estrogen, ovulation, CL development, production of progesterone, and if she does not conceive, repetition of the same events (usually) on a regular or somewhat predictable interval.

✓ Specific discussion of estrous physiology can be found in Section 5.

Estrous Detection and Teasing Program

✓ Inadequate or poor estrous detection or teasing methods are one of the major causes of reduced reproductive efficiency rates on many farms.

✓ The task is laborious, repetitive, time-consuming, and seldom enjoyed by farm personnel. The most skilled and interested people should be given the responsibility for this important breeding management activity. Consistency in observing each mare daily or every other day and an active or persistent and attentive stallion are key components to its success.

🔑 In pasture mating situations, this is the job of the herd sire.

✓ Two groups of mares should be the focus of most of the effort in the teasing program:

> Mares that have yet to be bred or inseminated.
>
> Mares that have been bred or inseminated at least 14 days previously and have exhibited diestrous behavior (i.e., teasing cold or out) during that period of time.

💣 Lactating mares require special attention as they frequently will fail to exhibit overt signs of estrus (i.e., tease hot or in) due to their protective behavior for their foal.

🔑 Mares that cycle normally, or exhibit regular intervals between periods of estrus, can be teased daily or every other day with one stallion.

✓ Mares that have erratic cycles or fail to show consistent signs of estrus may benefit from exposure to two different teasing stallions on a daily or every other day basis.

✓ Introduction of the stallion to the mare should occur as it does in the natural setting: allow or encourage a head-to-head approach of the stallion to the mare, allow him a slow interaction to judge her response, then progressively allow the stallion to move towards her tail. This will give the stallion, the mare, and the observing personnel time to accurately interpret the kind of interaction taking place.

🔑 Behavioral responses are important to observe and should NOT be rushed (Table 2-1).

Table 2-1
Signs of Estrus and Diestrus

POSITIVE SIGNS OF ESTRUS OR BEING IN HEAT	NEGATIVE SIGNS OF ESTRUS OR NOT IN HEAT
Tail-raising	Tail clamped tight
Leaning into teasing rail, or fence towards the stallion; not kicking or striking	Kicking, striking or biting at the stallion
Squatting to urinate	Indifferent attitude toward the stallion
"Winking" or rhythmic eversion of the vulvar lips exposing the clitoris	Failing to squat, urinate, or wink
Ears either forward or at half mast	Ears back

🗝 Flehmen response by the stallion (upper lip curl) is an indication the stallion has detected a pleasing odor or pheromone. It does not necessarily indicate that he has detected that the mare is in estrus.

💣 The teasing stallion must be under control in hand or in a teasing box. He needs to be interested in his task at hand, attentive and persistent, yet not overly aggressive as this may put some mares off. Shy mares, maiden mares, and wet mares typically do not respond to aggressive or overly attentive stallions (Figures 2-1 and 2-2) ⊙

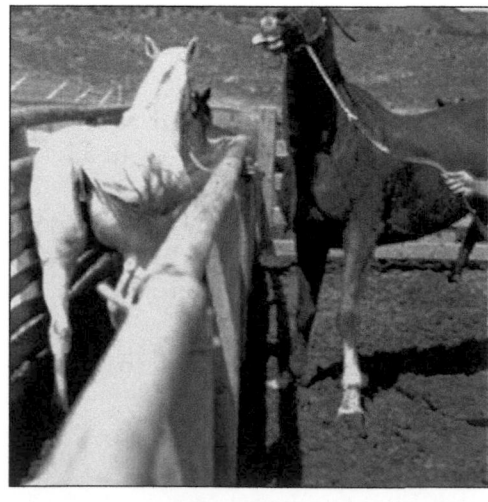

Figure 2-1 A stallion in hand teasing mares in a chute system at Colorado State University.

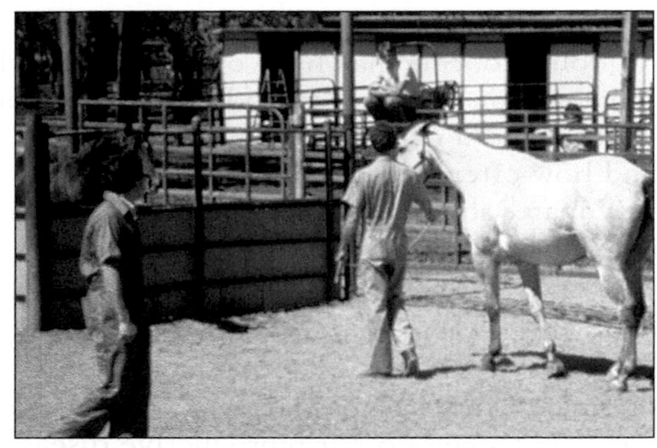

Figure 2-2 A stallion in a teasing box teasing mares in an adjoining dry lot at Texas A&M University.

✓ Pony stallions, some geldings, and occasionally a very masculine mare may sometimes be used to tease mares on farms where a stallion does not physically reside.

✓ Some mare owners are very attentive, know their mare's cycles, and can detect signs of their mare coming into estrus without the aid of teasing.

🔑 Squealing by the mare is a normal social response. At times a mare in estrus will squeal at the initial approach of the stallion, then 'break down' and show signs of being in heat. At other times, the same mare will squeal and then kick or strike and show no positive sign of estrus. ⦿ See CD of teasing demonstrations in a chute system (Videos 2-1 and 2-2).

✓ Mares that show signs of estrus should be scheduled for internal reproductive tract examination (i.e., vaginoscopy, rectal palpation and/or ultrasonography) to determine number, size, and location of follicles on her ovaries as well as other parameters to be discussed in Section 5 in this text.

💣 Mares will continue to tease hot, or show signs of estrus for 2-3 days AFTER ovulation occurs! Just because she is teasing in DOES NOT mean she is a candidate for breeding by natural service or artificial insemination. Good breeding management requires that the breeding be based on the development of the follicle(s), and breeding or insemination after ovulation occurs should be restricted to no more than 12 hours after the fact; 6 hours or less would be the optimum post-ovulation time that should be considered. Breeding mares too late after ovulation wastes stallion or semen resources and may predispose the mare to post-breeding endometritis which may interfere with embryonic survival if she happens to conceive.

✓ Mares showing no signs of heat should have a known reason for doing so. She may have ovulated more than 3 days ago as indicated by her records, and thus it is expected that she tease cold. If not, a reason needs to be identified. When to examine and how often is part of the art of breeding management. All new mares should be given an initial internal examination to determine where in their cycle they may be.

✋ Mares that continue to tease cold or out for more than 14 consecutive days, that are known NOT to be pregnant, that do NOT have evidence of active luteal tissue on either ovary (i.e., presence of a CL), that are in good body condition, and do not have evidence of other reproductive disease or pathology may benefit from teasing with an alternate stallion or estrous detection method (e.g., one-to-one across a tease rail, mare in paddock or stall next to the stallion). Other breeding management techniques for such mares will be covered in Section 6.

Behavior

✓ Breeding farm practices vary considerably around the world but, in general, impose considerable deviation from the natural environment and breeding behavior for both mares and stallions.

✓ Some of the modern horse husbandry practices are for safety and practicality, but many are more or less simply tradition.

✓ While most domestic horses breed successfully under intense domestic management, there is a considerable amount of sexual behavior dysfunction and/or sexual behavior related management and performance problems in horses under these conditions.

✓ Simple modification of husbandry to better model the natural social environment of horses while still considering safety of animals and handlers is often immediately effective in overcoming and preventing behavior problems.

✓ Standard breeding farm protocols include varying degrees of mare restraint. The restraint may interfere with normal horse to mare interactive behavior, receptive posture of the mare, the ability of the mare to adequately support the stallion, and to normally facilitate and accommodate intromission and thrusting.

✓ Play sexual behavior in young horses is another example of a normal frequent equine behavior that is commonly misunderstood as abnormal. Play sexual behavior with foal cohorts continues for fillies until maturity; with colts it is more frequent and continues into maturity as a bachelor stallion. Simply understanding that these interactions are normal and possibly important to development should reduce managers' concerns about the behavior and practices aimed at eliminating it.

✓ See Table 2-1 for a list of specific signs of estrus and diestrus.

Pasture Mating

✓ This is the most labor efficient and least expensive breeding management system in use.

Venereal disease transmission and injury to the animals are the greatest disadvantages.

✓ A stallion to mare ratio of 1:45 would be acceptable for most reproductively fit stallions with pasture breeding experience.

Conception rates for natural mating methods (both pasture and hand mating) range from 64-94% on a cumulative or seasonal basis.

> When reproductive records from 480 mares and 16 stallions were reviewed in one study, mean pregnancy rates ranged from 42-54% over a 48-day breeding period. More mares became pregnant in the last half of the breeding period (days 25 to 48) than the first half.

Hand Mating

✓ Hand mating is the most common method of breeding management in use for horses (Figure 2-3).

✓ Some of the advantages over pasture breeding include:

- Limiting the spread of venereal disease transmission
- Reducing the risk of injury to the animals involved
- Conserving stallion resources

Its disadvantages include:

- greater investment in time, labor, and equipment
- potential reduction in overall conception and pregnancy rate

Stallion to mare ratios in the range of 1:50 to 1:75 are typical. This is referred to as the stallion's book, or the number of mares he is scheduled to breed in a given season.

Question: Thoroughbreds are bred by live cover more than any

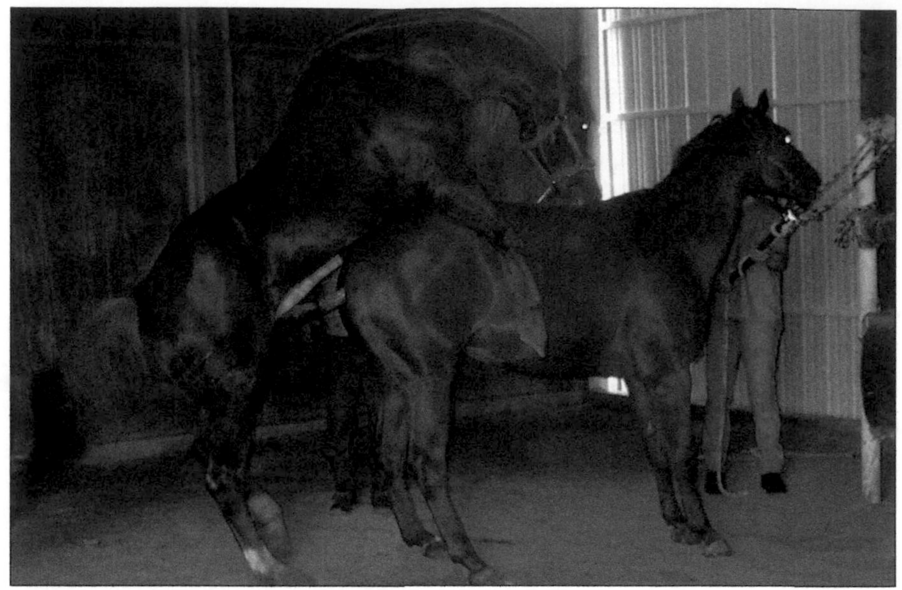

Figure 2-3 Live cover or hand mating on the farm.

other breed. What are the success rates associated with Thoroughbred hand mating programs?

Answer: Reproductive records from 639 Thoroughbred mares were analyzed, including information on the outcome of 2466 coverings in 1528 mare-years. Gestation length averaged 340.7 (± 0.24) days. Normal estrous intervals averaged 21.4 (± 0.1) days. There was no significant correlation between the lengths of successive estrous cycles in the same mare. Overall live foaling rate per covering was 39.8%. Fertilization failure and early embryonic death were 31.7%, while 2.3% of coverings resulted in abortion. The apparent late embryonic loss was 26.5%. The proportion of combined fertilization failure and early embryonic death decreased, and the apparent late embryonic loss increased from first to second to third services. Mares bred later in the season had better live foaling rates. Coverings carried out at the foaling heat had more fertilization failure and early embryonic death than those carried out at the next normal estrous. Lactating mares had apparently lower early embryonic death than non-lactating mares, but a higher incidence of infertility. Increasing age in the mare was accompanied by a decline in live foaling rate per covering.

Artificial Insemination (AI)

✓ This is the most technically advanced breeding management system for horses in popular use.

✓ Its advantages include:

- Nearly complete elimination of venereal disease transmission
- Elimination of the risk of injury to respective mare and stallion
- Greatest overall conservation of stallion resources
- Long distance breeding
- Expanded national and international markets
- Use of sex-sorted spermatozoa

✓ Its disadvantages include:

- Increased overall costs
- More intensive labor
- Greater requirement for equipment and facilities
- Greater level of technical expertise
- Certain breed registry restrictions limiting its use

🗝 Stallion to mare ratios of 1:250 are not uncommon.

✓ Conception rates for artificial inseminations have ranged from 67-98% on a cumulative or seasonal basis.

✓ Three common methods involving AI include:

- On the farm insemination with fresh, raw, or extended semen
- Transported fresh, extended, and cooled semen (Figure 2-4)
- Cryopreserved or frozen semen

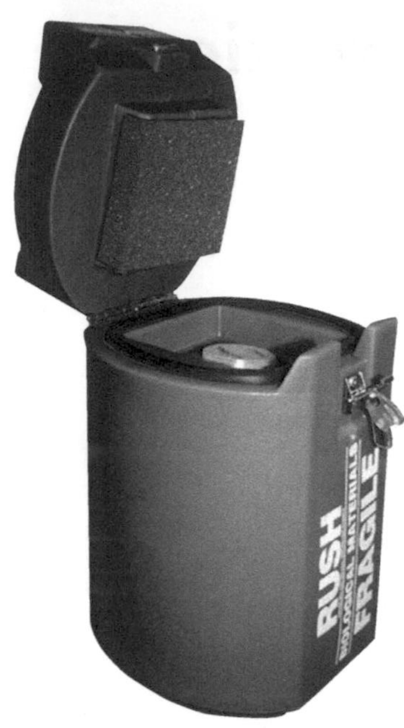

Figure 2-4 Stallion semen can be collected, diluted with an appropriate semen extender, cooled, and transported across the country or internationally to arrive within 24-48 hours of initial semen collection for AI in the mare that is ready to ovulate. (Equitainer II available from Hamilton Research Inc., http://www.equitainer.com/).

Question: I have talked with many clients about using frozen equine semen, but they have heard from friends and other horsemen that it is just not very successful. What can we expect from using frozen stallion semen in the mare?

Answer: In 1985, almost 32,000 mares were artificially inseminated using frozen semen in the northern provinces of China; 68% of these mares became pregnant. In Japan, the range in conception rate for frozen horse semen for 622 mares inseminated was 40-62% per cycle. Similar results are reported from work in the US with pregnancy rate ranging from 19-61% for single cycle inseminations. There are two primary considerations in the use of cryopreserved stallion semen for AI:

> There is a great deal of individual stallion variation as to how well his spermatozoa will survive the challenges of collection, processing for cryopreservation, storage, thawing, and insemination (Tables 2-2 and 2-3). Some stallions with excellent conception rates with AI on the

farm, or even with fresh, extended, cooled, and transported AI do not have respectable conception rates when their semen is inseminated following freezing and thawing.

The longevity (livability, viability) of frozen/thawed stallion semen once deposited into the mare's uterus is quite a lot shorter than when raw or fresh, extended, cooled, and transported semen is used for AI. This makes timing of the insemination in concert with the mare's ovulation much more challenging and critical to success. The window of opportunity (period of post-thaw viability) for some stallion's frozen/thawed semen may only be about 6 hours.

Table 2-2
Reproductive Efficiency Parameters for Cryopreserved Semen

PARAMETER	GROUP 1	GROUP 2	COMBINED
Number of stallions	100	6	106
Number of mares bred	641	235	876
1st cycle CR (%)	51.3	--	--
Seasonal PR (%)	71.9	85.5	75.6
Cycles per pregnancy	2.08	--	--

From Loomis, P.R. The equine frozen semen industry. *Anim Repro Sci* 68:191, 2001

Table 2-3
Reproductive Efficiency Parameters for Cooled and Frozen Semen

PARAMETER	COOLED	FROZEN DOMESTIC	FROZEN EXPORTED	FROZEN COMBINED
Number of stallions	16	96	10	106
Number of mares bred	850	340	536	876
1st cycle CR (%)	59.4	49.4	53.5	51.3
Seasonal PR (%)	74.7	65.6	81.9	75.6
Cycles per pregnancy	2.06	2.16	2.01	2.08

From Loomis, P.R. The equine frozen semen industry. *Anim Repro Sci* 68:191, 2001

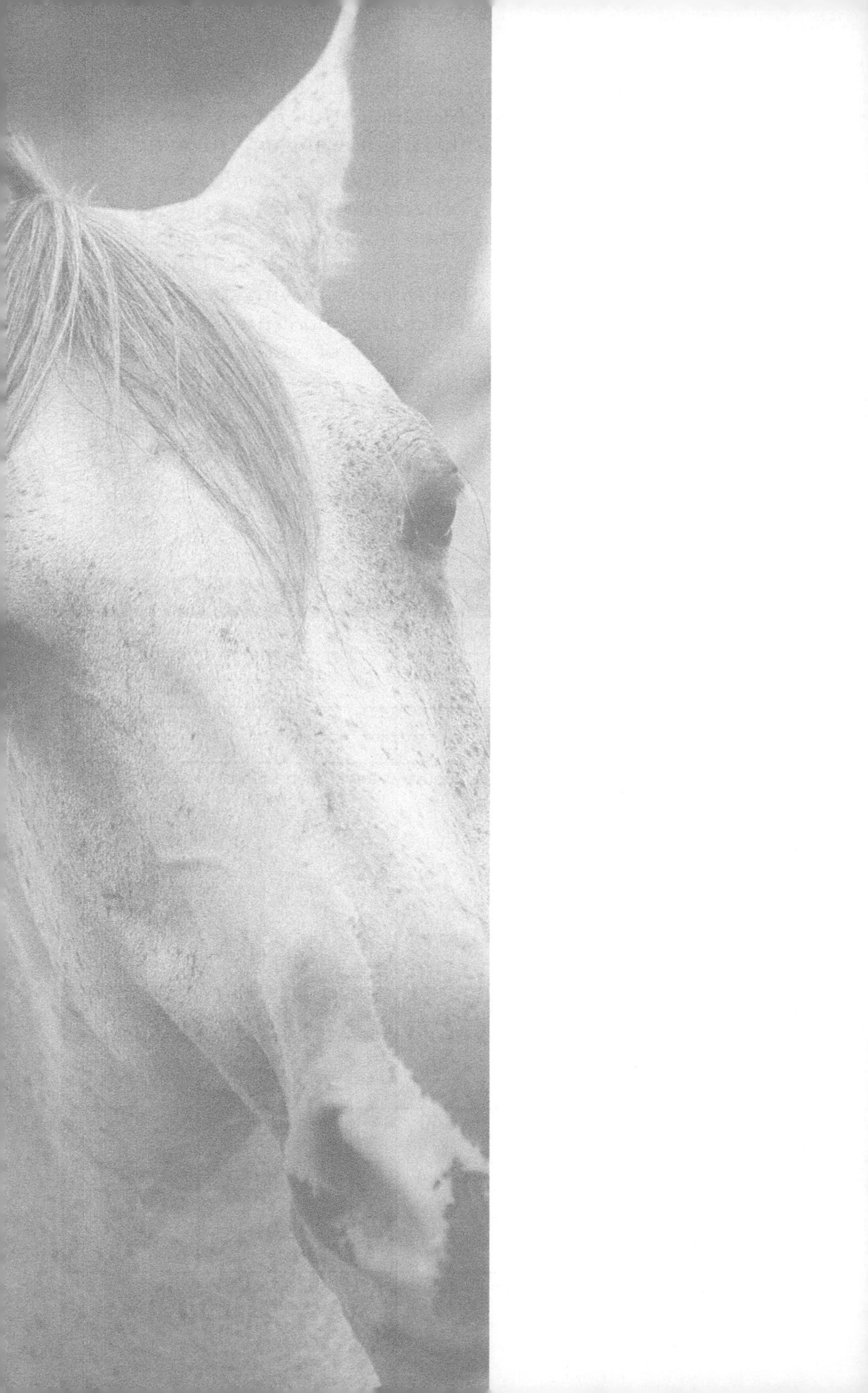

Section 3

Preventive Medicine Programs for Broodmares

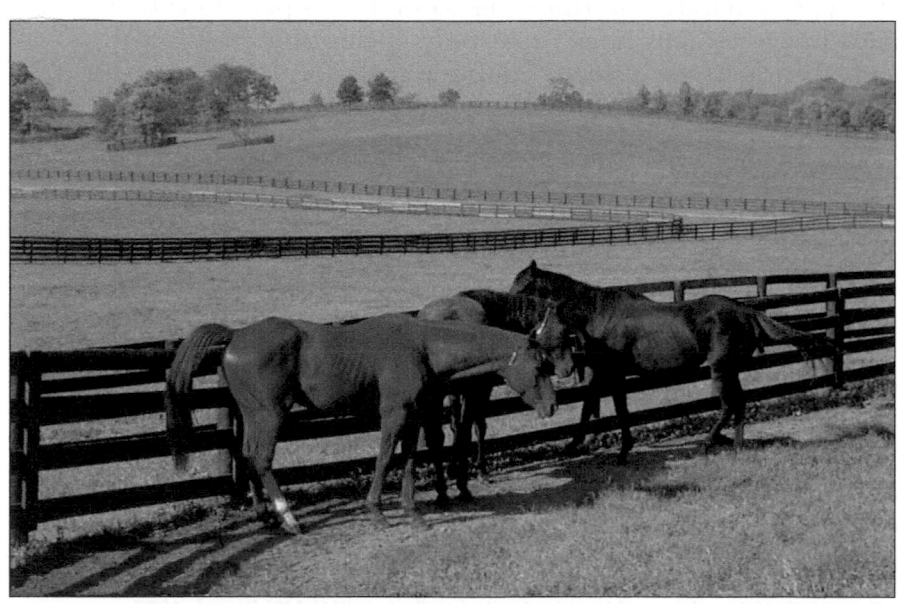

Introducing new animals to a group or herd can result in the introduction of a wide range of infectious agents such as parasites, viruses, and bacteria. One of the greatest threats to a horse's health is transmission of disease-causing organisms from another horse, whether by direct contact or through contact with contaminated aerosols, surfaces, equipment, vehicles, or the clothes and skin of people.

Biosecurity

Question: What is biosecurity?

Answer: Biosecurity procedures are management practices that limit exposure to disease. These practices can limit the spread of disease-causing organisms from one location to another or from one animal to another. Biosecurity is a concept used more and more in all animal health industries. It is an extension of preventive medicine programs which are designed to minimize introduction of disease into a group of animals. Biosecurity objectives include this as well as attempts to minimize the spread of disease from that group of animals.

🗝 One method of managing disease risk posed by introducing horses to an operation is isolation or quarantine of new arrivals for a period of time that exceeds the incubation period for disease onset.

✓ Approximately one-third (34%) of farm operations that added new resident horses routinely quarantined these new arrivals from their resident equine population.[1] As the size of the farm or operation increased, larger percentages of operations routinely quarantined new arrivals. For operations that routinely quarantined newly added horses, the average routine length of quarantine was 28.5 days.

✓ All new additions to the resident population of horses on any breeding farm or wherever pregnant broodmares reside must be quarantined for a minimum 30 days prior to their introduction to the resident herd. During this quarantine period, all horses should be evaluated for physical health and preventive measures implemented to be sure they are up-to-date on their routine immunizations.

✓ Preventing the introduction of new parasites into the pasture environment will also be a critical feature of the biosecurity program. New horses should be dewormed with a larvicidal dose of

[1] The USDA's National Animal Health Monitoring System (NAHMS) Report, 1998.

an effective anthelmintic to prevent introduction of potentially new anthelmintic-resistant strongyles. A treatment to prevent introduction of tapeworms to the pasture environment should also be incorporated.

✓ Depending on your area, it is also strongly advised, if not required by interstate movement regulations, to have all newcomers tested negative for equine infectious anemia (Coggins test) within 3-6 months prior to their arrival.

✓ During the quarantine procedure, any horse or any resident horse on pasture that develops soft stools or diarrhea should immediately be examined and assessed by fecal culture for the possibility of shedding *Salmonella*. Resident horses should go to quarantine until it is proven that they are not shedding this organism. While horse to horse fecal shedding of *Salmonella* is one potential source of this highly transmissible disease organism, remember that other contact sources can contribute to a disease outbreak with *Salmonella*; this can include contact with rodents or other domestic animals such as poultry, swine, or cattle. It is also possible that horses not showing signs of soft stool or diarrhea may be shedding the organism in the environment. Horses shedding the bacteria in feces may or may not show signs of illness.

✓ Not all *Salmonella* species will cause disease in the horse. The NAHMS Equine '98 study found 14 different serotypes of *Salmonella* species, several of which are not commonly associated with illness in horses. Fecal sampling results from the same NAHMS study showed a low prevalence of *Salmonella* shedding in U.S. horses. It was estimated that 0.8 percent of the horses shed *Salmonella*, and that at least one horse on 1.8 percent of operations shed the organism in its feces. The equine NAHMS study found that 1.4 percent of horses in the Southern region and 0.2 percent of horses in the Northern region were positive for *Salmonella* although these results were not statistically different

✓ Any horse with suspected upper respiratory infections (URI), like flu, rhino, or strangles, should be quarantined in a separate area of the farm or facility as far away from other horses as possible to prevent and minimize aerosol transmission of infectious agents between horses.

✓ Similarly, any horse with a low leukocyte count (low white blood cell count), fever, depression, inappetance, and soft stools or diarrhea should immediately be placed into quarantine.

🗝 Biosecurity procedures implemented for either URI or diarrhea include sanitary footbaths outside the stall door to prevent fomite transmission of agents throughout the barn. Examination and treatment of these horses should occur after the other horses have been examined and treated during the daily routine on the farm.

The quarantine stalls should be the last stalls cleaned each day and the bedding should be disposed of separately (bagged completely and transferred off the property to a disposal site where there is minimal risk of contaminating surface water or pastures).

Any and all halters, lead ropes, medical equipment, coveralls, gloves, etc., used in conjunction with the care and treatment of those horses in quarantine should be sanitized or sterilized or disposed of in a biosecure manner on a daily or more frequent basis as appropriate.

Stalls vacated by horses under quarantine should be thoroughly cleaned and disinfected using an effective protocol and left vacant for a minimum of 5 days between uses (Table 3-1).

Table 3-1
Suggested Sanitizing or Disinfecting Agents for Use in a Barn or Stall

Agent	Exposure time	Comments
Steam applied by pressure wash system	will vary by surface type; hard non-porous surfaces may only need a short contact time to kill most bacteria and viruses	An effective means of removing surface debris and organic material. Porous surfaces such as non-sealed wood may need a further application of a chemical disinfectant.
Glutaraldehyde based formulation (2%)	Follow manufacturer's recommendations	Caution should be exercised with all glutaraldehyde preparations when further in-use dilutions are anticipated.
Sodium hypochlorite (5.2% household bleach)	10-20 min; allow to soak into porous surfaces, then rinse residue	1:50 to 1:500 dilution range
Phenolic germicidal detergent solutions	< 10 min	Follow label instructions.
Iodophor germicidal detergent solution	< 10 min	Follow label instructions.
Quartenary ammonium germicidal detergent solution	< 10 min	Follow label instructions.

Immunizations

A standard vaccination program does not exist. Vaccination (immunization) is an aid to prevention of infectious diseases. Vaccination programs will not succeed without appropriate managerial practices.(Excerpt from AAEP, Guidelines for Vaccination of Horses. Jan., 2001.)

🗝 Immunizations are often thought of as the mainstay of the herd health or preventive medicine program; yet they are only one aspect of a much larger plan.

✓ Selection or design of a program must be adjusted to the needs and goals of the farm or its owner(s), as well as to the type(s), use, and ages of horses residing there.

✓ Components to consider when designing a specific program should include:

- The demographics of the population of horses to be protected
- Risk(s) of exposure to various infectious diseases in the respective area or region
- The severity or effects of the diseases to be included in the immunization program
- Availability, cost, and efficacy of vaccines under consideration
- Any potential adverse risk(s) associated with the use of such vaccines

💣 A summary of the immunization guidelines adopted by the American Association of Equine Practitioners is found in Table 3-2.

Table 3-2
Suggested Vaccination Schedule for Horses Recommended by the American Association of Equine Practitioners, 2001

The schedule below is a suggested vaccination schedule provided by the American Association of Equine Practitioners, and is based on generally accepted veterinary practices. Infectious disease control programs in conjunction with vaccination are important in maximizing the health, productivity and performance of your horse. Your veterinarian can help design a health management program to reduce exposure to infectious disease agents in your horse's environment and lessen the incidence of illness. Disease control programs should be tailored to your individual needs with consideration given to ages, types, activities and number of horses in your program. You should consult with your veterinarian regarding the specific needs of your horse.

Disease / Vaccine	Foals / Weanlings	Yearlings	Performance Horses	Pleasure Horses	Broodmares	Comments
Tetanus toxoid	From nonvaccinated mare: First dose: 3 to 4 mos. Second dose: 4 to 5 mos. Third dose: 5 to 6 mos.	Annual	Annual	Annual	Annual, 4 to 6 weeks prepartum	Booster at time of penetrating injury or surgery if last dose not administered within 6 Mos.
	From vaccinated mare: First dose: 6 mos. Second dose:7 mos. Third dose: 8 to 9 mos.					
Encephal-omyelitis (EEE, WEE, VEE)	EEE: (in high-risk areas) First dose: 3 to 4 mos Second dose: 4 to 5 mos Third dose: 5 to 6 mos.	Annual, spring	Annual, spring	Annual, spring	Annual, spring 4 to 6 weeks prepartum	In endemic areas booster EEE and WEE every 6 mos; VEE only needed when threat of

continued

						exposure; VEE may only be available as a combination vaccine with EEE and WEE.
Encephal omyelitis (EEE, WEE, VEE)	WEE, EEE (in low-risk areas) and VEE: From nonvacinnated mare: First dose: 3 to 4 mos. Second dose: 4 to 5 mos. Third dose: 5 to 6 mos. From vaccinated mare: First dose: 6 mos. Second dose: 7 mos. Third dose: 8 mos.	Annual, spring	Annual, spring	Annual, spring	Annual, spring 4 to 6 weeks prepartum	
Influenza	Inactivated injectable: From Nonvaccinated mare: First dose: 6 mos. Second dose: 7 mos. Third dose: 8 mos. Then at 3-mos. intervals	Every 3 to 4 mos.	Every 3 to 4 mos.	Annual with added boosters prior to likely exposure	At least semi-annual, with 1 booster 4 to 6 weeks prepartum	A series of at least 3 doses is recommended for primary immunization of foals
	From vaccinated mare: First dose: 9 mos. Second dose: 10 mos. Third dose: 11 to 12 mos. Then at 3-month intervals					

continued

Table 3-2 continued

Disease / Vaccine	Foals / Weanlings	Yearlings	Performance Horses	Pleasure Horses	Broodmares	Comments
Equine Herpesvirus (EHV-1, EHV-4)	Inactivated injectable: From Nonvaccinated mare: First dose: 6 mos. Second dose: 7 mos. Third dose: 8 mos. Then at 3-month intervals	Every 3 to 4 mos.	Every 3 to 4 mos.	Annual with added boosters prior to likely exposure	Pregnant mares: 5th, 7th, and 9th mos. of gestation and booster 4 to 6 weeks prepartum	A series of at least 3 doses is recommended for primary immunization of foals
	From vaccinated mare: First dose: 9 mos. Second dose: 10 mos. Third dose: 11 to 12 mos. Then at 3- month intervals					
Strangles	Injectable: First dose: 4 to 6 mos. Second dose: 5 to 7 mos. Third dose: 7 to 8 mos. (depending on product used) Fourth dose: 12 mos. Intranasal: First dose: 6 to 9 mos. Second dose: 3 weeks later	Semiannual	Optional: semi-annual if risk is high	Optional: semi-annual if risk is high	Semiannual with 1 dose of inacti-vated M-protein vaccine 4 to 6 weeks prepartum	Vaccines containing M-protein extract may be less reactive than whole-cell vaccines. Use when endemic conditions exist or risk is high. Foals as young as 6 weeks-of-

continued

						age may safely receive the in tranasal product by a 3rd dose should be administered before weaning.
Rabies	Foals born to non-vaccinated mares: First dose: 3 to 4 mos. Second dose: 12 mos. Foals born to vaccinated mares: First dose: 6 mos. Second dose: 7 mos. Third dose: 12 mos.	Annual	Annual	Annual	Annual, before breeding	Vaccination recommended in endemic areas. Do not use modified-live-virus vaccines in horses.
Potomac Horse Fever	First dose: 5 to 6 mos. Second dose: 6 to 7 mos.	Semiannual	Semiannual	Semiannual	Semiannual with 1 dose 4 to 6 weeks prepartum	Booster during May to June in endemic areas.
Botulism	Foal from vaccinated mare: 3-dose series of toxoid at 30-day intervals starting at 2 to 3 mos.-of- age	Not applicable	Not applicable	Not applicable	Initial 3-dose series at 30-day intervals with last dose 4 to 6 weeks prepartum. Annually thereafter, 4 to 6 weeks prepartum.	Only in endemic areas. A third dose administered 4 to 6 weeks after the second dose may improve the response of foals to primary immunization.

continued

Table 3-2 continued

Disease / Vaccine	Foals / Weanlings	Yearlings	Performance Horses	Pleasure Horses	Broodmares	Comments
Botulism	Foal from nonvaccinated mare: see comments					Foal from non-vaccinated mare may benefit from: 1) toxoid at 2, 4 and 8 weeks -of-age; 2) transfusion of plasma from vaccinated horse; or 3) antitoxin. Efficacy needs further study.
Equine Viral Arteritis	Intact colts intended to be breeding stallions: One dose at 6 to 12 mos.-of-age	Annual for colts intended to be breeding stallions	Annual for colts intended to be breeding stallions	Annual for colts intended to be breeding stallions	Annual for seronegative, open mares before breeding to Carrier stallions; isolate mares for 21 days after breeding to carrier stallion	Annual for breeding stallions and teasers, 28 days before start of breeding season; virus may be shed in semen for up to 21 days. Vaccinated mares do not develop clinical

continued

						signs even though they become transiently infected and may shed virus for a short time.
Rotavirus A	Little value to vaccinate foal because insufficient time to develop antibodies to protect during susceptible age	Not applicable	Not applicable	Not applicable	Vaccinate mares at 8, 9 and 10 mos. of gestation, each pregnancy. Passive transfer of colostral antibodies aid in prevention of rotaviral diarrhea in foals.	Check concentrations of immunoglobulins in foal to be assured that there is no failure of passive transfer.

*As with administration of all medications, the label and product insert should be read before administration of all vaccines.

†Schedules for stallions should be consistent with the vaccination program of the adult horse population on the farm and modified according to risk.

EEE = eastern equine encephalomyelitis; WEE - western encephalomyelitis; VEE = Venezuelan equine encephalomyelitis;

EHV-1 = equine herpesvirus type 1; EHV-4 = equine herpesvirus type 4.

Equine Influenza (A/ equi 1 and 2)

✓ One of the most common viral agents causing URI in horses of all ages, but horses 1 to 5 years of age are most susceptible.

✓ The risks of exposure are greatest on farms where horses come and go to shows, events, breeding farms, racetracks, and training facilities.

✓ Spread of the virus among groups of horses is by aerosol transmission from an infected coughing horse. Fomites such as feed and water buckets, grooming equipment, and tack may also contribute to its spread since the viral particles can survive in the environment for hours.

✓ Clinical signs include serous nasal discharge, epiphora, fever (usually greater than 103°F), anorexia, cough, and muscle stiffness or soreness.

✓ The protection offered with use of inactivated (killed) vaccines is short-lived; thus frequent booster immunizations are recommended for horses at high risk of exposure (every 90-120 days). The initial series in young immunologically naïve horses should be three doses separated by a 3 to 6 week interval.

✓ Pregnant broodmares should receive boosters 4-6 weeks prior to their due date.

✓ Foals can obtain passive transfer of protective antibodies directed against influenza when their dams have been appropriately immunized as above. Their initial series of influenza vaccinations should thus be delayed until 9 months of age to avoid competitive interference between passively acquired antibodies and the antigen presented in the vaccine.

✓ Foals born to dams not pre-immunized prior to foaling or that have had a failure of passive transfer may receive their initial series of influenza immunizations beginning around 6 months of age.

✓ A modified-live influenza (MLV) vaccine is available for intranasal administration. It is suggested that a single dose in a naïve horse may be protective for up to 6 months. This product is licensed for use in nonpregnant horses over 11 months of age.

Equine Herpesvirus (EHV1 and EHV4)

✓ Both EHV1 and EHV4 can cause URI (rhinopneumonitis "rhino") in horses.

✓ EHV1 causes abortion of virus-infected fetuses from infected mares, weak non-viable foals, and occasionally a neurologic posterior paresis to paralysis associated with a secondary vasculitis of the spinal cord and/or brain (myeloencephalopathy).

✓ The virus is spread by aerosol transmission from coughing infected horses, by direct contact with virus contaminated fomites, and through direct or indirect contact with virus infected placentae, placental fluids, and fetuses, or foals.

✓ Herpesviruses in many species including the horse have the ability to remain latent (dormant) in the animal causing no clinical signs. When stress occurs, a recrudescence of the infection occurs and the virus can then be spread to the environment and other horses.

✓ Repeated natural exposure to the virus does induce some immunity, as does the vaccine when used appropriately in the prevention of URI. Reliance solely on the vaccine to prevent either the abortigenic or neurologic forms of the disease has an inherent high degree of risk. Quarantine and isolation programs must be in place to further protect pregnant broodmares from introduction of new horses shedding the virus and thus minimize their risk of exposure.

✓ Pregnant mares should be vaccinated at the 5th, 7th, and 9th months of gestation with a licensed inactivated vaccine. Some practitioners recommend going off label, starting Herpesvirus immunization for pregnant mares at the 3rd month of gestation, and providing another booster at 11 months.

✓ Foaling mares should receive a prefoaling immunization 4-6 weeks prior to their due date to support colostral production of protective antibodies for their foals. This supports the recommendation for a booster at or around the 11th month of gestation.

✓ Barren mares and stallions should be vaccinated prior to the start of the breeding season.

✓ Initial immunization of foals that have had adequate colostral passive transfer of antibodies from a dam appropriately immunized prior to foaling should be delayed until the 6th month of age. The initial series is a 3 dose program of either a killed EHV1/EHV4 vaccine product or an MLV EHV1 product at 3-4 week intervals.

✓ Immunity is short-lived and thus young horses and others at high risk of exposure should be booster immunized at 3-4 month intervals.

✓ Immunization against EHV1 and EHV4 does not imply 100% protection against infection. But it may lessen severity of URI in younger horses.

✓ None of the available EHV1/EHV4 vaccine products to date have claimed any efficacy in prevention of the neurologic form of disease.

Equine Encephalitides (EEE, EWE, VEE and WNV)

✓ These viruses are all transmitted through mosquitoes. Mosquitoes and other blood-sucking insects are the vectors. The natural reservoir populations which harbor the viruses year round include birds and some small rodents. The risk of horse-to-horse or horse-to human transmission of the EEE or EWE through mosquitoes is extremely low due to the small amount of infecting virus particles present in the horse's blood system. The risk is somewhat greater with VEE.

✓ The mortality rate associated with EWE is about 50%. The mortality rate with EEE is nearly 90%. The mortality rate for VEE is between the two, but some horses infected with VEE develop subclinical disease, survive, and have a lasting immunity.

✓ The only vectors found to be associated with outbreaks of WNV in the United States since 1999 are mosquitoes. At least 30 species of mosquitoes have been found positive for WNV, although several of those species are likely not involved in active transmission of the virus from bird-to-bird or from bird-to-mammal.

✓ Horses are affected by WNV much more often than any other domestic animal. Many horses infected with WNV do not develop any illness, but of horses that become ill about one-third (33%) die or need to be humanely destroyed. Other livestock and poultry do not commonly show any illness if infected with WNV.

⊙ The mortality rate associated with WNV, the newest of the encephalitides introduced into the US has been variable. For the latest information visit the web site maintained by the United States Agriculture Department, Animal and Plant Health Inspection Service (USDA APHIS):
http://www.aphis.usda.gov/oa/wnv/2001_summary.html

⊙ The total number of equine cases of illness caused by WNV confirmed at the USDA's NVSL or reported by state officials from Jan to Oct 2002 was 9036. There was an increase of 1574 cases reported over one 7 day interval. New cases were reported from 36 states. The USDA APHIS Summary Report: Update on the Current Status of West Nile Virus is found at: http://www.aphis.usda.gov/oa/wnv/wnvstats.html.

✓ Vaccination with a killed product for EEE, EWE, WNV or the MLV for VEE provides some protective immunity against these diseases. But vector control must also be part of the overall biosecurity program.

✓ The initial series of immunizations should be 3 doses 3 to 4 weeks apart. Adults will respond well to a 2 dose initial series.

✓ In endemic areas, a booster vaccination for EEE is recommended at 6 month intervals. All are administered as annual boosters after the initial immunization schedule.

✓ Pregnant mares should be booster vaccinated 4 to 6 weeks prior to foaling to provide colostral antibodies in support of passive transfer to foals.

⊙ The WNV vaccine to date has not received licensed approval for use in pregnant mares or stallions. Check with the manufacturer for an update prior to its administration. Web site information: http://www.wyeth.com/products/ahp_products/animal_health.asp

The protection provided by the vaccination must be present prior to the peak of the mosquito season.

Equine Arteritis Virus Infection (EAV, EVA)

Many horses affected with this virus show no symptoms or signs of the disease.

✓ Naïve horses may show fulminant clinical signs with fever, anorexia, depression, lethargy, swelling of the face and/or eyelids, edema of the extremities, epiphora, and serous nasal discharge. Occasionally young animals may succumb from pneumonia, secondary to infections with EAV. Pregnant mares may abort. Stallions infected with EAV may shed the virus in their semen, sometimes for life.

Prevention programs include a combination of serologic surveillance and immunization only of known serologically negative horses with an MLV vaccine approved for use in the U.S. (ARVAC™, Ft. Dodge Laboratories, Ft. Dodge, IA)

Vaccination of nonpregnant mares and stallions is considered safe and effective. However, vaccine virus may shed from these individuals for a period of up to 21 days, thus they should be in a quarantine or isolation situation during this time period to prevent inappropriate transmission to pregnant mares.

✓ A single dose of the approved MLV vaccine is sufficient for both primary and annually administered booster immunizations.

Rabies

✓ Horses can become infected with the rabies virus through the bite of an infected rabid animal.

✓ The disease once contracted is invariably fatal.

✓ Vaccination is the key to prevention and control must also include programs to suppress if not eliminate the disease from wildlife and other domestic animals in or around the farm and region.

✓ Killed products are used in horses, with an initial dose given at 3-4 months of age for foals that did not receive colostral passive transfer from a protected dam, and at 6 months of age for those that did. Their booster immunization should occur at 1 year of age, and then is repeated annually.

✓ None of the licensed products are approved for use in pregnant mares.

✓ MLV products for use in horses against rabies are not approved for use in the U.S.

Rotavirus

✓ Diarrhea in foals is a common problem. Rotavirus infection may contribute to up to 50% of the foal diarrheas in some areas.

🗝 Vaccination of the dam 4-6 weeks prior to foaling in an effort to stimulate colostral antibody production against the virus, and thus passively protect the foal once it has consumed a sufficient quantity of colostrum has been recommended in endemic areas.

🗝 A vaccine against the Rotavirus "A" strain is commercially available in the U.S. It does not provide cross-protection against the Rotavirus "B" strain. A 3 dose series is required at each pregnancy at 8, 9, and 10 months of gestation.

✓ There is no evidence to suggest that use of the vaccine in foals will have any protective benefit as a primary immunostimulant.

Equine Strangles (*Streptococcus equi* subsp. *equi*; i.e., equine distemper)

🗝 This is primarily a disease of juvenile horses although older horses are known to become severely infected as well.

🗝 Transmission is by direct contact with nasal secretion (mucopurulent), or abscess discharge. Indirect transmission can occur through contaminated fomites.

✋ *Strep equi* can survive in the environment for up to 3 months when it is sheltered from direct sunlight, dessication, or disinfectants.

🗝 Affected horses present with high fever (102 to 106°F). anorexia, nasal discharge which turns mucopurulent, and may develop internal lymph node abscessation under the jaw, around the pharynx, and potentially deeper in the abdominal cavity.

🗝 *Strep equi* subsp. *zooepidemicus* can cause similar signs, although usually such infections do not involve lymph nodes to the point of abscessation.

🗝 Bacterins, an inactivated sub-unit (M-protein) vaccine for intramuscular administration, and a modified live bacterial vaccine for intranasal administration are available for use in prevention and control programs. None have proven highly effective in preventing infections, although they may lessen the severity of disease once the infection starts.

💣 Whole cell bacterins cause significant reactions and muscle soreness at the site of injection and may precipitate abscess development at such sites.

✓ Vaccination against strangles is not routinely recommended, except in very endemic areas or on farms where an outbreak has occurred.

💣 Within 2 to 4 weeks following natural or vaccine-induced exposure to the antigens of *Strep equi*, some horses are at risk of developing purpura hemorrhagica, an immune-mediated vasculitis syndrome. This may be life threatening.

Anthrax

✓ A serious and rapidly fatal septicemia caused by the vegetative form of the bacterial organism, *Bacillus anthracis*.

✋ Vaccination of horses against anthrax is indicated only in endemic areas.

✓ There is currently not a licensed approved vaccine for use in horses in the U.S.

💣 The Sterne's strain licensed for use in cattle has been used in some situations to prevent the disease in horses. This is a non-encapsulated live spore vaccine and thus serious precautions must be exercised in storage, handling, and administration of the product.

Potomac Horse Fever (PHF), Equine Monocytic Ehrlichiosis (EME)

✓ This is caused by the organism *Ehrlichia risticii.*

🔑 The disease is seasonal (late spring to early fall), regional (occurring primarily in the Eastern U.S.), and does not seem to be transmissible between horses.

✓ Trematode parasites of fresh water snails seem to be its natural vector in transmission.

✓ Clinical signs vary greatly but most present with high fever (104-107°F), lethargy, anorexia, reduced intestinal peristalsis, mild to watery profuse diarrhea, colic, dehydration, and laminitis.

✓ Vaccination against the disease is suspect or questioned as field evidence does not support its benefit of use.

✓ In endemic areas, an initial 2 dose series is administered 3-4 weeks apart, and booster vaccinations are recommended by some practitioners as frequently as every 3-4 months.

✋ If vaccination against PHF is elected as part of the preventive medicine plan, it should be strategically timed to induce maximal vaccine response prior to the summer months where greatest risk of exposure occurs.

✓ Vaccines currently approved for use in horses are licensed to include stallions and pregnant mares.

✓ Since foals are seldom affected, their primary immunization does not need to start before 5-6 months of age, regardless of whether the mare was pre-immunized prior to foaling, or not.

Equine Protozoal Myelitis / Myeloencephalitis (EPM)

✓ The agent of concern in this disease is the protozoa *Sarcocystis neurona.*

🗝 In the natural life cycle (yet to be entirely resolved) this organism uses two intermediate hosts to complete its development. The definitive host is considered to be the opossum, and one or more intermediate hosts (striped skunk, armadillo, domestic and feral cats) are also required to propagate the organism. Contamination of the organism's infective sporocysts in fecal deposits from infected host into the environment results in the horse becoming victimized as an innocent bystander.

🗝 The horse is a dead end host (i.e., does not transmit the infection to other animals).

🗝 Many horses show evidence of being seropositive (maybe as high as 50% of the population in some areas, exposure and/or infection). But a far less number actually exhibit clinical signs of the disease.

✓ The disease once initiated is progressively debilitating to the neurologic system of the horse. Early signs may present as a mild lameness. Other affected horses may initially show signs of abnormal upper respiratory function or even seizures.

🗝 The variability in clinical signs is due in part to the fact that the organism can induce damage sporadically within the grey or white matter of the brain, brainstem, or spinal cord.

✓ A vaccine is commercially available and licensed as an aid in prevention of this disease. Its use has been limited to endemic areas, and its efficacy is still open to question.

Tetanus Toxoid

💣 No horse should live his or her life without being immunized with tetanus toxoid. It is a simple vaccination to perform and very cost effective.

✓ Tetanus is very often fatal. The organism *Clostridium tetani* is ubiquitous on farms and in and around horses.

✓ Although not considered contagious or infectious, its inclusion in the preventive health care program for all horses is standard.

✓ Nonvaccinated horses respond well to an initial 2 dose series 3-6 weeks apart. Annual boosters are given thereafter, although protective antibodies may persist for as long as 5-7 years after proper immunization.

✓ Pregnant mares should be booster vaccinated with tetanus toxoid 4-6 weeks prior to foaling. Foals from such mares having received adequate passive transfer through her colostrum do not start their active immunization schedule against tetanus until at least 6 months of age.

✓ Foals not receiving adequate colostral protection should begin their series at 3-4 months of age and receive 3 doses 3-6 weeks apart rather than the 2 doses recommended above.

✓ Tetanus antitoxin (TAT) is reserved for use in injured nonvaccinated horses. Administration of 1500 IU will provide passive protection for up to 2-3 weeks.

A small number of horses have developed serum sickness (fatal hepatic failure) 2-4 weeks after administration of TAT.

It is acceptable practice to administer TAT and tetanus toxoid at the same time (using separate syringes) in nonvaccinated and injured horses, or foals born to mares not having been pre-immunized before foaling, and to foals that have had a failure of passive transfer.

Botulism

✓ Horses have been known to suffer from three different forms of disease when exposed to the botulinum toxin or infected with the organism *Clostridium botulinum:* Toxicoinfectious botulism or shaker foal syndrome (type B toxin)

Forage-based toxicity from exposure while grazing

Wound botulism when directly infected with the organism

Botulism toxin is the most potent organism-produced toxin known.

✓ Clinical signs include muscle weakness progressing to paralysis, inability to masticate and swallow, and potentially death by asphyxiation.

There are eight known toxin types produced by the organism; types B and C are most often associated with equine cases.

✓ A toxoid against the type B toxin is licensed for use in endemic areas of the US.

✓ Pregnant mares are vaccinated with the type B toxoid prior to foaling with a 3 dose series 4 weeks apart timed so that the third dose is given within the final 4-6 weeks of gestation.

✓ Mares previously vaccinated are given a single annual dose 4-6 weeks prior to foaling.

✓ Foals from previously nonimmunized dams or that have had a failure of passive transfer may be vaccinated with the type B toxoid as early as 2 weeks of age, with boosters at 4 and 8 weeks of age.

✓ In endemic areas or farms, foals born to mares that have been immunized prior to parturition should start their active immunization schedule at 2-3 months of age and receive a 3 dose series 4 weeks apart.

Cross-protection of immunity between type B toxin antigens and the other toxins (including type C) produced by this organism does not occur. Yet there are no other vaccines currently approved in the US other than for protection against the *Clostridium botulinum* toxin type B.

Parasite Control

✓ While anthelmintic drug usage has been the mainstay of parasite control in horses for many decades, minimizing exposure to infective parasitic larvae through pasture hygiene (a nonchemical approach) must be included in the preventive health care program.

✓ Heavy dependence on chemicals has led to widespread drug resistance to at least the benzimadazole class of anthelmintics.

✓ There is a need to attack equine parasites in the environment. General guidelines include:

Pick up and dispose of manure on a regular basis (at least twice weekly).

Mow and harrow pastures regularly to break up manure piles and expose parasite eggs and larvae to the elements.

Rotate pastures by allowing other livestock such as sheep or cattle to graze them, thereby interrupting the life cycles of equine parasites.

Group horses by age to reduce exposure to certain parasites and maximize the deworming program geared to that group.

Keep the number of horses per acre to a minimum to prevent overgrazing and reduce the fecal contamination per acre.

Use a feeder for hay and grain rather than feeding on the ground.

Remove bot eggs quickly and regularly from the horse's haircoat to prevent ingestion by clipping the affected areas or by using a scraper, a bot egg knife, or a warm water sponge.

Rotate deworming agents, not just brand names, to prevent chemical resistance.

🗝 The most common parasites of concern in the control program include:

Large strongyles (bloodworms)

Small strongyles (cyathostomes)

Ascarids (roundworms)

Pinworms

Bots

Tapeworms

Threadworms

Lungworms

✓ One of the most under-utilized tools in an effective parasite control program is the fecal examination. This simple diagnostic process can identify the specific parasites infecting a horse. Rarely are the worms themselves visible in the manure. Fecal eggs per gram counts (EPG) are a helpful indication of the type and the degree of parasite infestation on a farm or within a herd, as well as useful determinants to assess the efficacy of anthelmintic usage.

🗝 Horses at different ages and stages have varying needs concerning parasite control. Young foals are especially susceptible to ascarid (roundworm) infestation, and may benefit from deworming at 30 day intervals until they build some natural resistance. Older horses turned out on a large pasture might do well on a semi-annual schedule. And some owners may prefer to have their horses on a continuous control program whereby the horse is given a daily dose of dewormer through a feed additive.

✓ Most often, different classes of broad spectrum drugs such as ivermectin, pyrantel pamoate, and oxibendazole are rotated every two months throughout the year.

✓ Another approach is the seasonal program, based on the local climate and parasite populations. For example, a seasonal program may call for a deworming at the start of grazing season, with dewormers rotated every two months while the horse is on pasture. At the end of the grazing season, a dewormer effective against bots should be used.

🗝 Ivermectin alone is highly effective against bots. It should be given in the spring after bot eggs are produced, and again in the late fall to remove any bots picked up during the grazing season.

💣 Many parasitologists and pharmacologists feel that it is only a matter of time before ivermectin and moxidectin-resistant cyathostomes emerge. This is particularly important in that the small strongyles, or cyathostomes, have become recognized as the most common internal parasites of horses in developed countries.

🗝 Tapeworms can cause intermittent colic. A horse may have tapeworms even if no eggs are found in a fecal test. Pyrantel pamoate is effective against tapeworms, and many equine veterinarians recommend giving it once a year at double the label dose for effective removal of tapeworms.

💣 Moxidectin, a newer anthelmintic on the market, or high doses of fenbendazole are effective against encysted small strongyles. Moxidectin is also reported to be effective against roundworms, small and large strongyles, pinworms, bots, hairworms, and stomach worms. It has been shown to be effective against strongyles for up to three months in adult horses, a month longer than the standard two-month dosing interval.

💣 Horse owners should be cautioned that Moxidectin suppresses roundworms for only 6 to 8 weeks. Because foals are highly sensitive to roundworm infections, horses under 2 years of age that are given moxidectin should be dewormed at 2 month intervals. Foals less than 4 months of age should not be treated with moxidectin.

Nutrition

Horses evolved as grazing animals and do best when fed a diet high in, if not completely composed of, forages. Forages are grasses or legumes, fresh or dried (e.g., hay) and are also referred to as the roughage portion of the diet. Horses can have their roughage requirements met by feeding at least 1% of their diet as forage.

✓ Nutritional requirements for the horse are based on two basic needs--maintenance and performance (i.e., athletic work, growth, lactation, etc.)

✓ Grains (also known as concentrates) are higher in digestible energy density than roughages by 50-60% and are fed primarily when energy demands exceed those met by the forage provided.

✓ Fats or oils (vegetable or grain-derived) have 2.25 times the amount of digestible energy per pound than grains or concentrates. They have been used successfully to increase the energy density of the horse's diet when fed at no more than 10-15% of the total ration or diet by weight. When doing so, an additional amount of vitamin E should be supplemented as well.

✓ Body condition scoring (Table 3-3 and Figure 3-1) is a useful tool to evaluate the adequacy of the nutritional program, and to monitor its success over time.

Management of the broodmare should be to maintain above average body condition (6 on a scale of 1 to 10).

Mares foaling in better than average body condition and maiden and barren mares at or above average body condition conceive sooner than mares in less than average body condition.

✓ Obese mares or those with body condition score greater than 8 tend to have more difficulty conceiving. Some obese mares may warrant investigation of hypothyroidism.

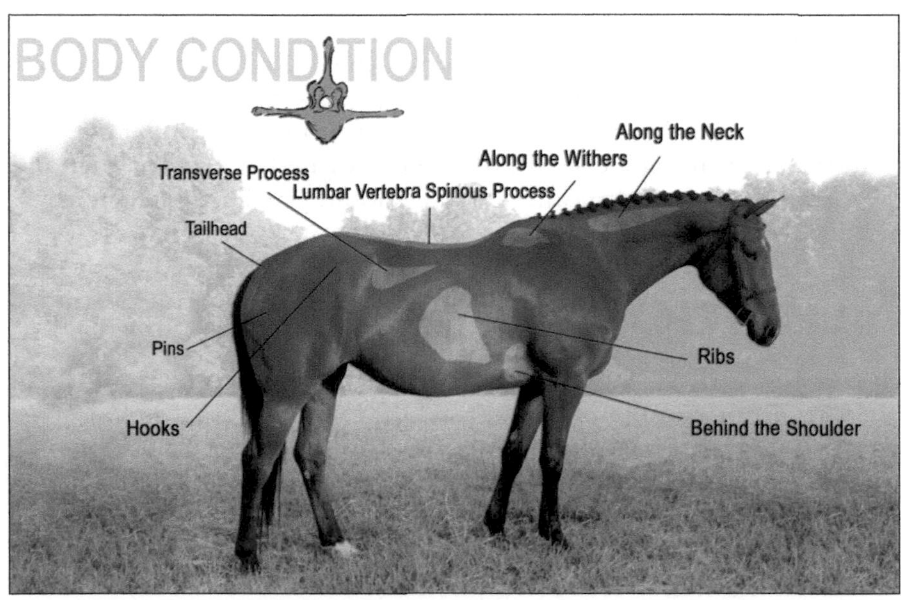

Figure 3-1 Body condition scoring system for the horse: areas of the body to evaluate.

Table 3-3
Body Condition Scoring System for the Horse: Descriptive Parameters

Condition Score	Neck	Whithers	Loin	Tailhead, Pins & Hooks	Ribs	Shoulder
1 Poor	Bone structure easily noticeable. Animal extremely emaciated, no fatty tissue can be felt.	Bone structure easily noticeable.	Prominent spinous processes.	Tailhead and hooks and pins project prominently.	Ribs project prominently.	Noticeable bone structure on shoulder.
2 Very Thin	Neck faintly discernible. Animal emaciated.	Withers faintly discernible.	Slight fat covering over base of spinous processes. Transverse processes of lumbar vertebrae feel rounded. Spinous processes are prominent.	Tailhead and hooks and pins are prominent.	Ribs prominent.	Shoulder faintly discernible.
3 Thin	Neck accentuated.	Withers accentuated.	Fat built up about halfway on spinous processes. Transverse processes cannot be left.	Tailhead prominent, but individual vertebrae cannot be visually identified. Hook bones appear rounded, but easily discernible. Spinous processes easily discernible. Pin bones not distinguishable.	Slight fat cover over ribs. Ribs easily discernible.	Shoulder accentuated.

continued

Table 3-3 continued

Condition Score	Neck	Whithers	Loin	Tailhead, Pins & Hooks	Ribs	Shoulder
4 Moderate to Thin	Neck not obviously thin.	Withers not obviously thin.	Spinous process (ridge) along back.	Tailhead prominence depends on conformation, fat can be felt around it. Hook bones not discernible.	Faint outline of ribs discernible.	Shoulder not obviously thin.
5 Moderate	Neck blends smoothly into body.	Withers appear rounded over spinous processes.	Back is level.	Fat around tailhead beginning to feel spongy.	Ribs cannot be visually distinguished but can be easily felt.	Shoulder blends smoothly into body.
6 Moderate to Fleshy	Fat beginning to be deposited.	Fat beginning to be deposited.	May have slight crease down back.	Fat around tailhead feels soft.	Fat over ribs feels spongy.	Fat beginning to be deposited.
7 Fleshy	Fat deposited along neck.	Fat deposited along withers.	May have crease down back.	Fat around tailhead feels soft.	Individual ribs can be felt, but noticeable filling between ribs with fat.	Fat deposited behind shoulders.
8 Fat	Noticeable thickening of neck. Fat deposited along inner buttocks.	Area along withers filled with fat. Fat deposited along inner buttocks.	Crease down back.	Fat around tailhead very soft.	Difficult to palpate ribs.	Area behind shoulder filled in flush.
9 Very Fat	Bulging fat.	Bulging fat.	Obvious crease down back.	Bulging fat around tailhead. Fat along inner buttocks may rub together. Flank filled in flush.	Patchy fat appearing over ribs.	Bulging fat.

Adapted from: Lawrence, LA: Nutrient requirements and balancing rations for horses. VA Coop Ext, Publ. No. 406-473, July, 1996.

✓ Micromineral nutrient requirements for broodmares do not differ from that of the mature nonpregnant horse until late in gestation and during lactation (Table 3-4).

✓ Sodium levels are below minimum requirements in most all feedstuffs. Salt is a basic element of all nutrition programs whether it is supplemented as a component in a complete feed or as a block or loose mix granule in the pasture or stall.

✓ Good quality forages usually provide adequate calcium and phosphorus to meet maintenance needs.

To be sure that the ration provided is adequate a complete forage analysis is highly recommended.

✓ During the first 8 months of gestation, the nutrient requirements of broodmares are only slightly above that recommended for maintenance. More than 60% of the final weight gain and growth of the fetus occurs in the last trimester of gestation.

✓ Milk production (lactation) greatly increases most nutrient requirements of the mare. The mare has the ability to produce up to 3% of her body weight in milk during her first 90 days of lactation, and another 2% during the next 60 to 100 days.

✓ Water is a nutrient and is a requirement at all times. A good clean source of water should be available at all times (free choice), preferably kept at or around 40°F.

Table 3-4
Nutrient Concentrations in Total Diets for the Mature Horse and for the Pregnant Broodmare

Nutrient	Mature Horse	Preg- 9 mos	Preg- 10 mos	Preg- 11 mos
Digestible energy, Mcal/kg[1]	2.00	2.25	2.25	2.40
Crude protein, %[2]	8.0	10.0	10.0	10.6
Calcium, %	0.24	0.43	0.43	0.45
Phosphorus, %	0.17	0.32	0.32	0.34
Vitamin A, IU/kg	1830	3710	3650	3650
Vitamin D, IU/kg	300	600	600	600
Vitamin E, IU/kg	50	80	80	80

From Nutrient Requirements of Horses, 5th Rev Ed., Washington, D.C., Nat Acad Press, 1989.
[1]Values are per kg feed and assumes concentrate contains 3.3Mcal/kg and hay contains 2.0 Mcal/kg dry matter.
[2]Percent on a dry matter basis.

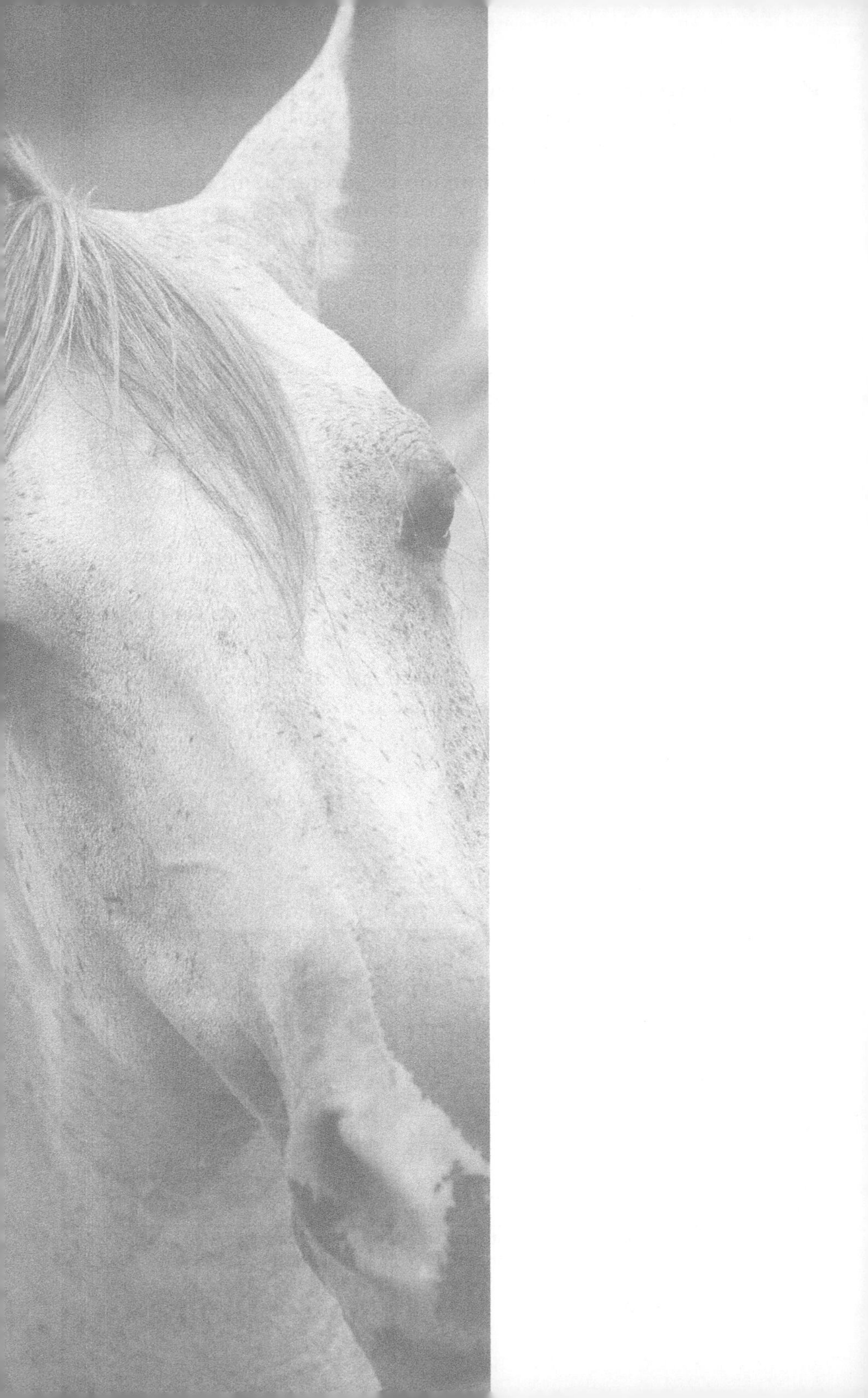

Section 4

Anatomy and Physiology

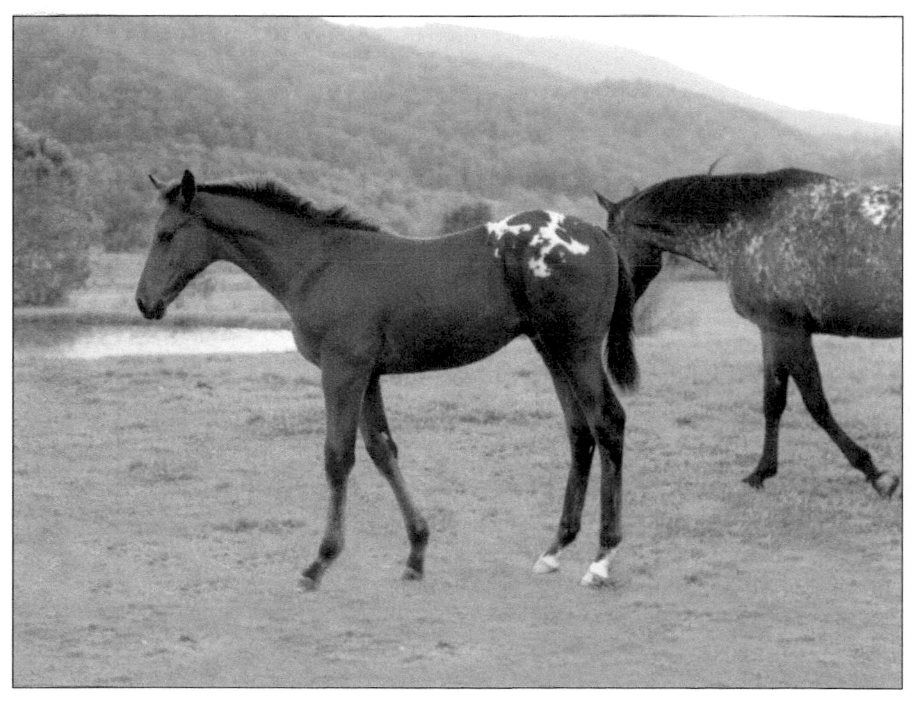

Perineal Conformation and Anatomy

✓ The external genitalia of the mare are comprised of the perineum and the labia of the vulva.

✓ The perineum is defined as the body wall encompassing the outlet of the pelvis and surrounding the urogenital tract outlet, and the distal rectum and anus.

✓ The limits of the perineum are the base of the tail and coccygeal muscles dorsally, the sacrosciatic ligaments and semimembranosus muscles laterally, and the ischial arch and origin of the udder ventrally (Figure 4-1).

✓ Nerve supply to the muscles of this area is contributed by the deep perineal nerves. Caudal rectal and pudendal nerves, arising from sacral segments 3 to 5, provide motor and sensory fibers to the anal sphincter and dorsal perineal areas. The ventral and lateral areas of the perineum are provided with sensory fibers from branches of the caudal cutaneous femoral nerve emanating from sacral segments 1 and 2.

☞ Such a nerve distribution pattern accounts for the variable response to attempted anesthesia of the perineum by epidural route.

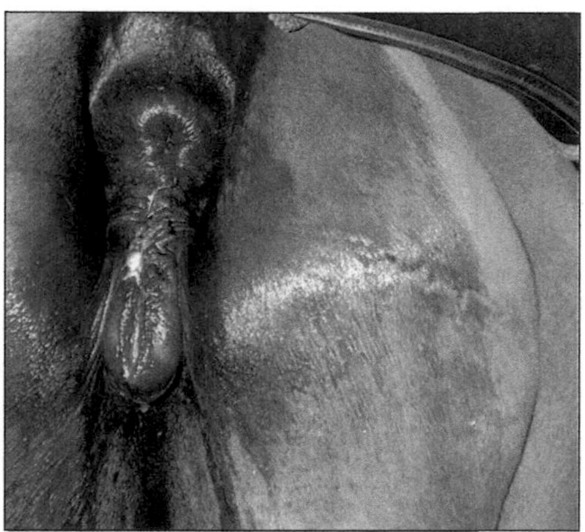

Figure 4-1 Perineum of the mare.

Vulva, Vestibule, and Vagina

✓ The vulva is defined as that portion of the genital tract common to both the urinary and reproductive systems. It includes the two labia, the clitoris and its associated sinuses, fossa, and glans.

✓ The vulva is ventral to the rectum and anus, dorsal to the pelvic floor, and is flanked laterally by sacrosciatic ligaments and the semimembranosus muscles on each side.

✓ The external opening of the vulva, or vulval cleft, is typically 12 to 15 cm in length and is confined by the labia.

✓ The sharp junction of the labia near the anal sphincter is referred to as the dorsal commissure. The confluence ventrally is more rounded, surrounds the clitoral area, and is termed the ventral commissure.

✓ The vulva, in its normal position, drapes over the ischial arch of the pelvis in such a manner that the level of the dorsal commissure of the labia should be at, or ventral to, this bony structure (Figure 4-2).

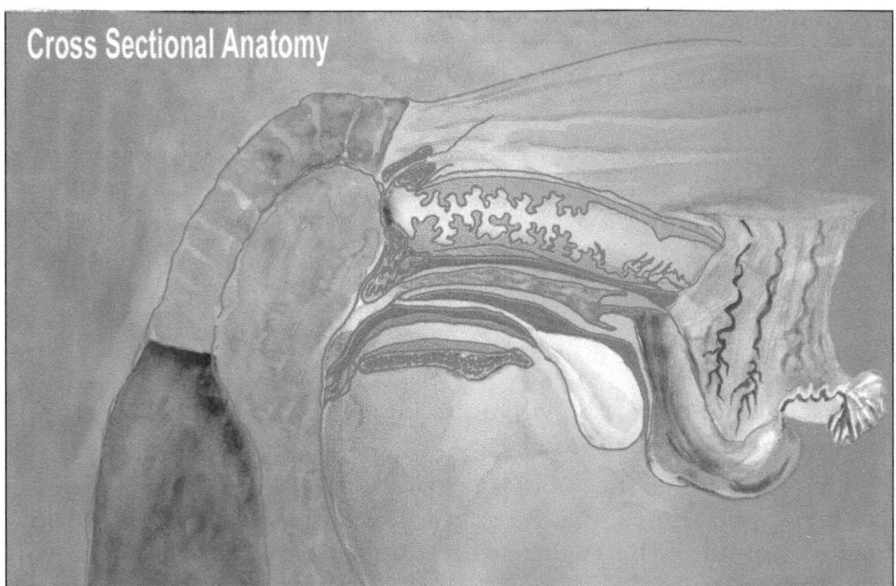

Figure 4-2 Cross-sectional diagram of the relationship of the vulva to the ischial arch and pelvis of the mare.

✓ The elastic thin usually pigmented skin of the labia is richly supplied with sebaceous and sweat glands. Deep to the skin lie the skeletal muscle fibers of the constrictor vulvae, and on each side are also the smooth muscles of the clitoral retractor muscle. Dorsally the constrictor vulvae muscle is continuous with the caudal part of the external anal sphincter muscle.

The clitoris is the homologue of the penis. The glans clitoris is approximately 2.5 cm in diameter and is covered by wrinkled creased skin (Figure 4-3). It is surrounded laterally and ventrally by the clitoral fossa which at its deepest portions can be 7 to 8 mm deep. A transverse frenular fold of integument covers the glans dorsally. A singular median clitoral sinus and two lateral frenular sinuses are present with various depths just ventral to the transverse frenular fold. The body of the clitoris (corpus) is about 5 cm long and is attached to the ischial arch by two crura. It contains erectile tissue, the corpus cavernosum clitoridis, which is homologous to the corpus cavernosum penis.

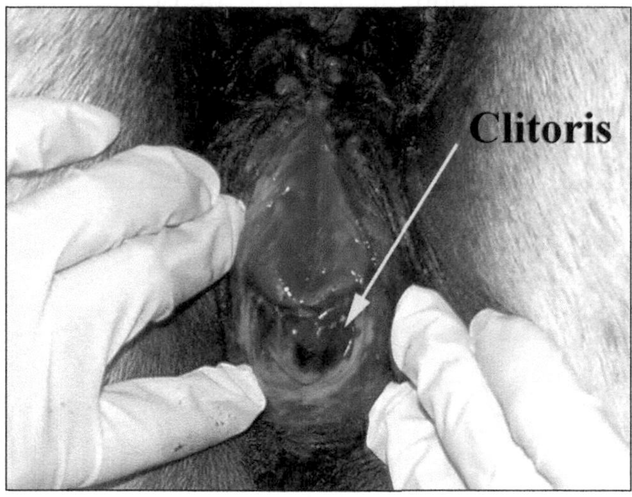

Figure 4-3 Clitoris of the mare.

✓ Vascular supply to the vulva, its labia, and the clitoris is by the internal pudendal vessels.

✓ The vestibule is the tubular portion of the vulva connecting the labia with the vagina. Its cranial extent is at the level of the transverse fold of the vagina, which lies just rostral and dorsal to the urethral orifice.

✓ The dorsal wall of the vestibule is, by comparison, short with respect to its sloping ventral wall. The normal configuration of the vestibular vault should have a ventrodorsal slope in the rostral direction.

✓ The vestibular bulb is a mass of erectile tissue approximately 3 by 7 cm. It is related laterally with the constrictor muscle of the vestibule, medially by a comparatively darker region of vestibular mucous membrane, and located just rostral to the labia.

✓ The thin-walled vagina ends caudally at the transverse fold above the external urethral opening where it is contiguous with the vestibule.

✓ The transverse fold is a remnant of the hymen, which partitioned the vestibule from the vagina proper during embryogenesis. The transverse fold marks the line of merger between the cranial portion of the reproductive tract, which is of mesodermal origin, and the caudal portion, which is of ectodermal origin.

✓ The vagina may be up to 20 cm in depth. The vaginal fornix is an annular recess formed by the joining of the cranial vaginal walls and the vaginal portion (external os) of the uterine cervix (Figure 4-4).

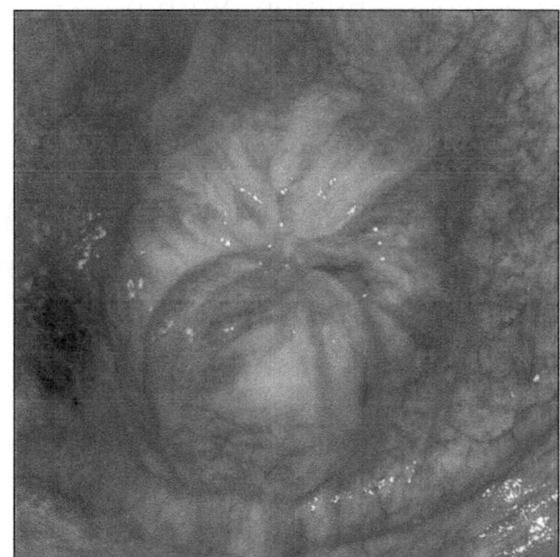

Figure 4-4 Anterior vaginal fornix and external os of the mare.

✓ The vaginal mucous membrane is aglandular. The longitudinal folds of the vaginal mucous membrane are effaced with distension of its lumen. Its tissues are fibroelastic to allow passage of the foal at parturition. It is surrounded by loose collagenous connective tissue which contain numerous sympathetic ganglia, a venous plexus, and varying degrees of adipose tissue.

✓ The portion of the cranial vagina that is covered by peritoneum is related inversely with the amount of fullness in the rectum and urinary bladder. Peritoneum reflects from the rectum onto the anterior-dorsal vaginal wall and forms the rectogenital pouch. Peritoneum also reflects from the urinary bladder to the anterior-ventral and lateral walls of the vagina forming the vesicogenital pouch.

When the rectum and bladder are relatively empty, sufficient peritoneum (about 8 to 10 cm) reflects onto the vagina to allow entry into the rectogenital pouch surgically via the colpotomy procedure. Caudodorsally the vagina is separated from the rectum by the rectovaginal septum.

Vaginal venous varicosities arising within branches of the middle hemorrhoidal vein occasionally develop within the vaginal wall, more commonly in the dorsal region just cranial to the transverse fold or near remnants of the hymen. These can be a source of a bloody vaginal discharge or frank hemorrhage during late gestation.

The vaginal mucous membrane and vaginal wall are devoid of nervous sensation. With no skeletal muscle present, no motor innervation is supplied. There are multiple sympathetic ganglia present within the vaginal wall supplied by branches of renal, aortic, uterine, and pelvic plexuses.

Uterus, Uterine Tubes, Ovaries, and Adnexa

Cervix

✓ The uterine cervix is the constricted thick-walled muscular extension of the uterine body that is 5.0 to 7.5 cm in length. Its distal end projects caudally into the anterior vagina.

✓ Longitudinal mucosal folds run the length of the cervical canal; these are continuous with endometrial folds of the uterine body and end caudally at the protruding portion of the cervix in the anterior vaginal space.

✓ A fold of mucosa may extend ventrally from the external cervical os to the floor of the vagina; this is referred to as a frenulum.

✓ To a variable extent, there may also be a dorsal frenulum that suspends the external os from the roof of the anterior vaginal vault.

✓ The mucosa of the cervix is grossly more pale than that of the uterus proper. Tubular gland openings do not project through the cervical mucosal surface as seen in the endometrium.

✓ The cervical mucosa is highly folded and fern-like in appearance. Its epithelium has both ciliated and mucus-secreting cells. The cervical wall contains a significant amount of collagenous connective tissue and a sphincter of smooth muscle derived from the inner layer of the myometrium. The cervix is within the respective rectogenital and vesicogenital pouches.

Uterus

✓ The uterine body and horns are typically "Y" or "T "shaped. The body is cylindrical and is partly situated in the abdominal cavity, and partly within the pelvic cavity (Figure 4-5).

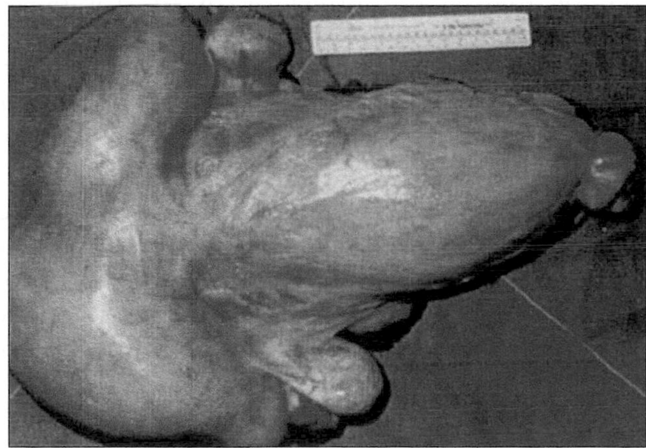

Figure 4-5 Mares reproductive system at post mortem examination demonstrating uterus filled with purulent material (pyometra).

✓ The body is flattened dorsoventrally and averages 18 to 20 cm in length. The endometrial surface is similar to that of the uterine horns but with fewer tubular gland openings on the surface.

🗝 A short intrauterine, or median, septum marks the bifurcation between right and left horns at their juncture with the uterine body. The intercornual ligament on the serosal surface is less prominent in the mare as compared with that of the cow and should not be used as a means of retracting the uterus during rectal examination.

✓ The uterine horns are located entirely within the abdominal cavity. Their lengths range from 20 to 25 cm in the nonpregnant state and are usually symmetrical in shape; however, they tend to lose their symmetry with successive pregnancies. The serosal surface is comprised of visceral peritoneum, or perimetrium, which on the dorsal, or attached, border is continuous with the two peritoneal sheets of the mesometrium, also called the broad ligament.

✓ The uterine horn diameter is typically smaller near the blunt tip and progressively enlarges toward the junction with the uterine body.

✓ The broad ligament attaches the uterine body and horns to the abdominal and pelvic walls. It originates in the lateral sublumbar region (from the 3rd or 4th lumbar to the 4th sacral vertebra) and the lateral pelvic walls, and extends to the dorsal, or attached, border of the horns and the lateral margins of the uterine body.

✓ The mesometrium is continuous with the perimetrium of the free, or unattached, surface of the uterine horns. The double sheet of peritoneum of the mesometrium encloses vessels, nerves, connective tissue, lymphatics, loose collagenous tissue, adipose tissue, and sheets of smooth muscle that are continuous with the outer longitudinal layer of smooth muscle of the myometrium.

✓ The ureters are situated along the parietal margins of the broad ligaments. The round ligament of the uterus is located in a fold along the lateral margin of the mesometrium. This homologue of the gubernaculum testis originates above the blunt end of the horn where it forms a large round appendix; it then passes caudoventrad to the internal inguinal canal where it blends with the parietal peritoneum.

✓ The lumen of the uterus is practically obliterated by surrounding intra-abdominal pressures. Five to ten longitudinal endometrial folds occupy the collapsed lumen from body to uterotubal junction (Figure 4-6).

✓ Vascular supply to the uterine horns on each side comes from three sources: the uterine branch of the vaginal artery, or caudal uterine artery (from the internal pudendal artery); the uterine artery (from the external iliac artery); and the uterine branch of the ovarian artery, or cranial uterine artery. The main venous drainage of the uterus is by way of the uterine branch of the ovarian vein.

🗝 The uterus does not receive sensory innervation.

Figure 4-6 Ultrasonogram of a cross-section of one uterine horn demonstrating endometrial folds.

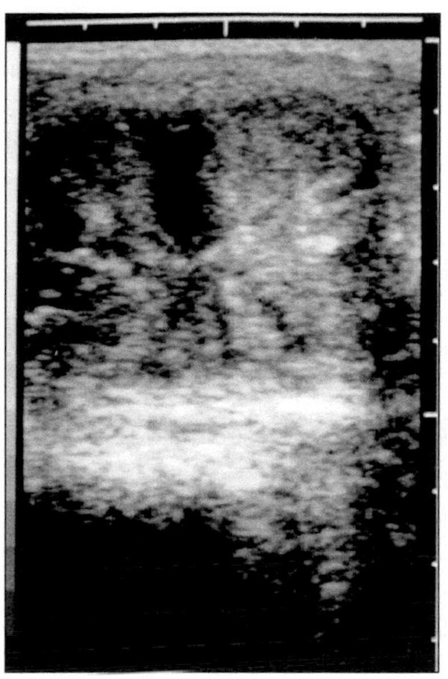

✓ The epithelial layer of the endometrium is simple columnar, with cuboidal to tall cells dependent upon the stage of the estrous cycle. Branching tubular endometrial glands extend from their openings at the epithelial surface through the compact layer of the lamina propria to the spongy layer located just beneath the inner circular layer of smooth muscle of the myometrium (Figure 4-7).

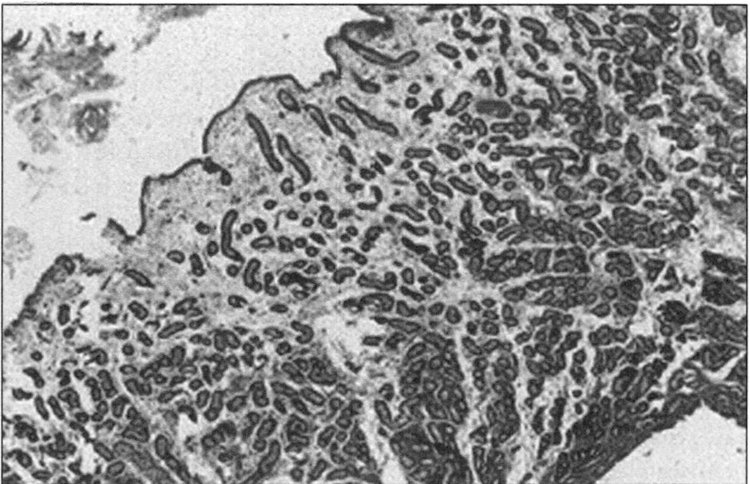

Figure 4-7 Histologic cross-section of the endometrium showing glandular structures in the stratum compactum and stratum spongiousum.

🗝 Internally, the lumen of each horn ends at the ostium of the uterine tube. A small papilla is formed at this opening by a sphincter of circular smooth muscle; this creates an effective valve in the mare preventing entry of uterine luminal contents into the uterine tube (Figure 4-8). ⊙

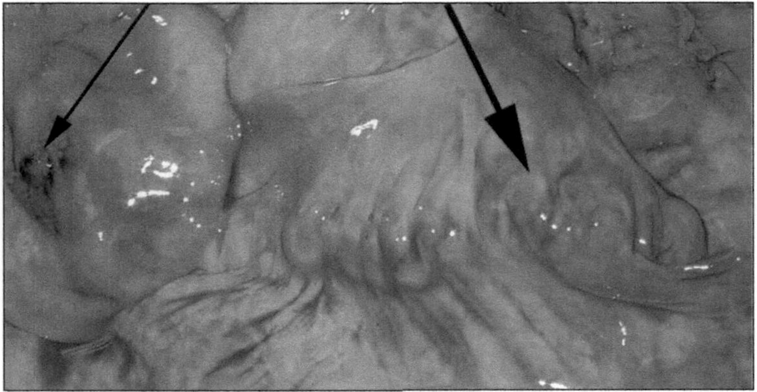

Figure 4-8 The ostium of the uterine tube ending in the papilla at the tip of this dissected uterine horn tip (small arrow). The oviduct (uterine tube) has been injected with India ink to darken its path as it courses through the mesosalpinx (large arrow).

Oviducts

✓ The oviduct (salpinx, uterine tube, or Fallopian tube) is divided into three parts: the isthmus, the ampulla, and the infundibulum.

✓ The oviduct ranges from 20 to 30 cm in length with the ampulla comprising half of the total.

✓ The transition from ampulla to isthmus is gradual. The ampulla has an expanded lumen that is about 6 mm in diameter. This is in comparison to the isthmus proper which has a diameter of 2 to 3 mm. The ampulla is also highly tortuous whereas the isthmus is relatively straight.

✓ The abdominal ostium of the oviduct, in the center of the infundibulum, is the dividing point between the infundibulum and the ampulla.

✓ The infundibulum is funnel shaped. Its margin consists of irregular folds called fimbriae. At the rostral edge of the infundibulum, some fimbriae are attached to the cranial pole of the ovary forming the cranial edge of the ovulation fossa. The remaining fimbriae spread over the ventral aspect of the ovary to cover the ovulation fossa (Figure 4-9).

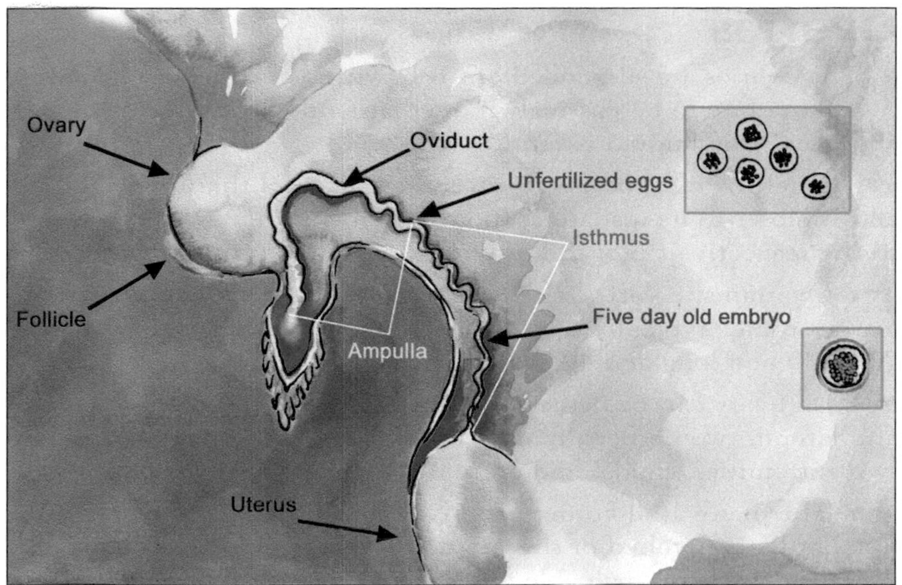

Figure 4-9 Illustration of the relationship of the ovary, oviduct, and mesovarium.

🗝 The ovarian bursa of the mare is a pouch lined by peritoneum. It extends from the ovulation fossa caudally to the cranial aspect of the uterine horn. Its lateral bounds are formed by the uterine tube and its mesosalpinx. Its medial bounds are formed by the proper ligament of the ovary which is a fold of the broad ligament.

🗝 An unusual phenomenon in mares is the retention of nonfertilized ova in their oviducts. This occurs either in or near the ampullary-isthmus junction in both bred and nonbred mares.

🖑 Granulosa cells near the time of ovulation secrete a basophilic sticky mucoid substance which invests the ovum and corona radiata cells. This substance is released with the ovum at ovulation and enters the uterine ostium. The ovum becomes separated from this mass by 2 days post-ovulation.

🖑 Retention of cumulative nonfertilized ova, globular oviductal masses, and the presence of non-occlusive salpingitis remain as potential problems to investigate in barren mares that fail to conceive while demonstrating otherwise normal or acceptable reproductive findings on breeding serviceability examinations.

Ovaries

✓ The ovaries are suspended entirely within the abdominal cavity and are free to be passively moved around within the abdomen, to a limited extent.

✓ The left ovary is usually located more caudal than the right and is closer to its ipsilateral kidney. The distance from the ovary to the respective tip of the ipsilateral uterine horn also varies.

🗝 Ovarian size varies with season of the year and stage of the estrous cycle. Typically they are bean- or kidney-shaped, and are 70 to 80 mm long and 40 to 60 mm wide.

✓ Each ovary can be described as possessing two surfaces, medial and lateral, two borders, free and attached (or mesovarial), and two extremities, caudal and cranial.

🗝 The mesovarial border is convex and situated dorsally. The free border is notched or sharply concave and is located ventrally. This depression, palpable upon rectal palpation, is the ovulation (ovarian) fossa (Figure 4-10). ⊙

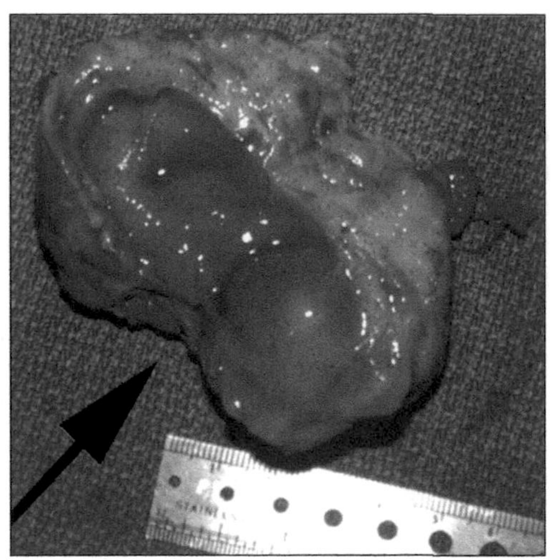

Figure 4-10
The ovary of the mare showing the ovulation fossa.

✓ The cranial pole (tubal extremity) is rounded and is related to the fimbriae of the infundibulum. The caudal pole (uterine extremity) is also rounded and is connected to the uterine horn by the proper ovarian ligament.

✓ The ovaries are suspended in the abdominal cavity by the cranial portion of the broad ligament, or mesovarium. Within this structure course vessels, nerves, and smooth muscle fibers that reach the ovary along its dorsal or mesovarial border.

✓ The convex surface of the ovary is therefore its hilus, that portion of the organ where vessels and nerves enter and depart. The visceral peritoneal covering of the ovary is loosely attached with deposits of adipose tissue and loose connective tissue intervening between the peritoneal investiture and the ovary itself.

The histologic structure and embryogenesis of the equine ovary is unique among domestic animals. The mature ovary has a peripheral collagenous connective tissue vascular zone (or medulla) surrounding a central parenchymatous zone (or cortex) containing developing and atretic ovarian follicles, corpora lutea, and corpora albicantia.

The germinal epithelium of the horse is confined to the ovulation fossa of the adult ovary. The parenchymatous zone emerges at the ovarian fossa and during folliculogenesis, Graafian (or maturing) follicles move toward the fossa where ovulation occurs in all cases.

✓ Sympathetic nerve fibers to the ovaries, uterine tubes, and uterus are supplied from plexuses in renal, aortic, uterine, and pelvic locations. These fibers accompany arterial branches to the respective areas. The internal spermatic nerve accompanies the ovarian artery and innervates the ovary, uterine tube, and cranial portion of the uterine horn.

Adnexa

Adnexal structures that may occasionally be found in or near the internal genital tract of the mare are often fluid-filled embryonic vestiges.

✓ Fimbrial cysts (hydatids of Morgagni) are common in mares. They frequently are pedunculated and histologically are lined with ciliated columnar epithelium, indicating that they are of Mullerian duct origin.

✓ Fossal cysts may also be found in the region of the ovulation fossa. These are similar to fimbrial cysts and their impact on fertility of the mare is open to question. Large numbers of small cysts, or large cysts few in number, may obstruct the normal ovulatory function of infundibulum and ovulation fossa.

✓ Tubal (paraovarian) cysts are remnants of the mesonephric duct system. These may be found in the mesosalpinx or mesovarium and be from 2 to 50 mm in diameter.

✓ Cysts forming in the cranial group of mesonephric tubules are epoophoron.

✓ Those forming more caudally are paroophoron.

Physiology of Ova Production and Fertilization

The equine female begins life with a pool of about 40,000 primordial follicles.

Folliculogenesis

✓ Folliculogenesis in the mare is a physiologic event that can be divided into three phases; recruitment, selection, and dominance.

🗝 Following puberty, or with entry into each new physiologic breeding season following anestrus, when an adequate amount of circulating gonadotrophins becomes available in the circulation, follicles are recruited from the dynamic pool of small follicles (i.e., < 10 mm).

✓ Small antral follicles are continuously growing and regressing independent of the hormonal events taking place in the mare throughout her lifetime.

✓ A group of growing preantral follicles becomes responsive to, and then dependent on, gonadotrophins, especially follicle stimulating hormone (FSH), for their continued growth and differentiation. This is termed recruitment.

✓ Recruited follicles grow in synchrony until eventual selection occurs, whereby one or more dominant and several subordinate follicles continue to grow.

✓ The selected dominant follicle(s) continues to grow to a large diameter (e.g., > 30 mm) while the subordinate follicles undergo atresia.

🗝 The vast majority of follicles that develop beyond 1 mm in diameter are destined to undergo atresia.

✓ Mares have one or two major episodes or waves of follicle development during the estrous cycle. In interovulatory cycles in which two waves occur, the first wave that develops is referred to as the secondary wave. Its emergence takes place in late estrus or early diestrus.

✓ The wave that contributes the dominant follicle(s) that will ovulate in the subsequent estrus is referred to as the primary wave. Its emergence is at mid-diestrus.

🗝 The dominant follicle(s) that develops in the secondary wave may occasionally ovulate under the progesterone dominant period of diestrus; if not, regression without ovulation occurs.

✓ Follicles that reach dominance produce factors that directly or indirectly cause regression of the other follicles in its own wave and further prevent emergence of additional follicles of a new wave.

✓ Dominant follicles require gonadotrophins for their continued development, synthesis and secretion of estradiol, and eventual ovulation.

✓ Estradiol is the key hormone for promoting folliculogenesis and for triggering the physiologic events necessary for reproductive behavior.

✓ The dominant follicles must therefore possess an enhanced capacity for estradiol synthesis and secretion over other follicles. Such a capacity involves the action of both FSH and luteinizing hormone (LH) on follicular theca and granulosa cells.

✓ Granulosa cells in preantral follicles contain FSH receptors but do not develop receptors for LH until antrum formation. Beginning at the preantral stage, theca cells possess receptors for LH but never develop FSH receptors.

✓ Follicular fluid within the antrum contains numerous factors other than steroid hormones that are potential intragonadal modulators of folliculogenesis (e.g., insulin, prolactin, prorenin, relaxin, oxytocin, inhibin, activin, hypoxanthine, and adenosine). Most of these factors are inhibitory to follicular function and may be integral products secreted by each follicle that are necessary to cause atresia.

🗝 The predominant ovarian event is atresia. It is estimated that more than 99% of all follicles in the human ovary become atretic. In the mare, between 50 and 75% of the follicles at a given time, regardless of size, are undergoing degeneration or atresia.

✓ A long-loop feedback system between a dominant follicle and the pituitary gland exists to orchestrate the selection process. Follicular fluid contains inhibin and estradiol, both of which suppress follicle stimulating hormone (FSH) secretion. FSH enhances inhibin and estradiol synthesis in granulosa cell cultures in vitro. These form the basis for a classical long-loop negative feedback system.

✓ The ability of the dominant follicle to survive in a hormonal milieu that is suppressive to growth of other follicles, may be explained in part by the fact that estradiol, which markedly enhances FSH and luteinizing hormone (LH) action, is found in significantly greater concentration in the antral fluid of dominant follicles (other subordinate follicles) (Figure 4-11). ⊙

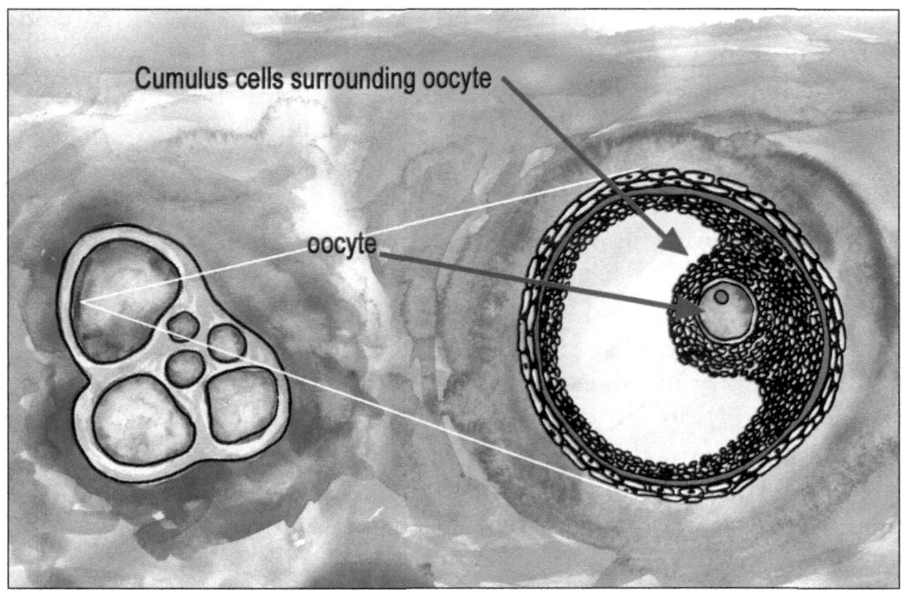

Figure 4-11 Illustration of the ovary with a large preovulatory follicle and enlargement depicting the ova within the antrum.

Oogenesis

✓ Oogenesis is the process of development of the ovum within the follicle. It begins with oogonia, which originate from primordial germ cells in the embryo.

✓ Some oogonia enter the first stage of meiosis in the fetal gonad, beginning around day 80 of gestation. These resulting cells are then 1º oocytes and are arrested in the first stage of meiosis (prophase I). Some of these 1° oocytes at mid-gestation become associated with surrounding cells and form primordial follicles.

✓ At birth, tens of thousands of primordial follicles containing 1° oocytes form the pool of gametes for the reproductive life of the mare. They remain arrested until follicle atresia occurs, or until stimulated within pre-ovulatory follicles by a surge of LH to continue their meiotic reduction division.

✓ Following the peak of the ovulatory LH surge during estrus, the nuclear membrane of the arrested 1° oocyte disintegrates signaling the resumption of meiosis. During the first division, the chromosome numbers are halved and the resulting cell is then the 2° oocyte. The discarded half-complement of chromosomes is sequestered inside the first polar body, which is retained within the zona pellucida of the 2° oocyte. The 2° oocyte is then arrested during the second meiotic division in metaphase II.

✓ The approximate diameter of the equine 2° oocyte is 125μ, devoid of zona pellucida and corona radiata (Figures 4-12 and 4-13).

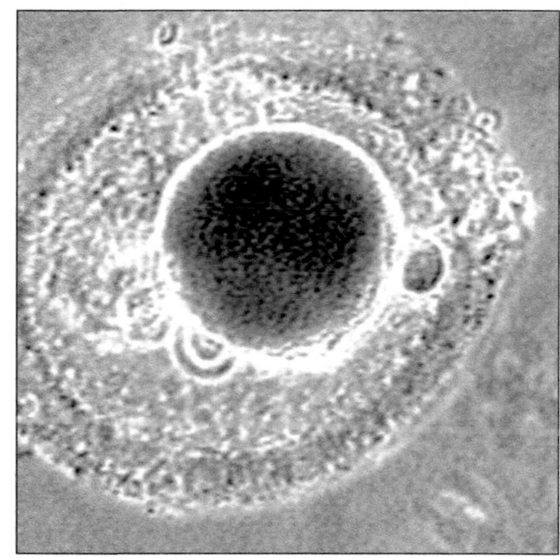

Figure 4-12
The equine secondary oocyte with polar body shown at 3 o'clock.

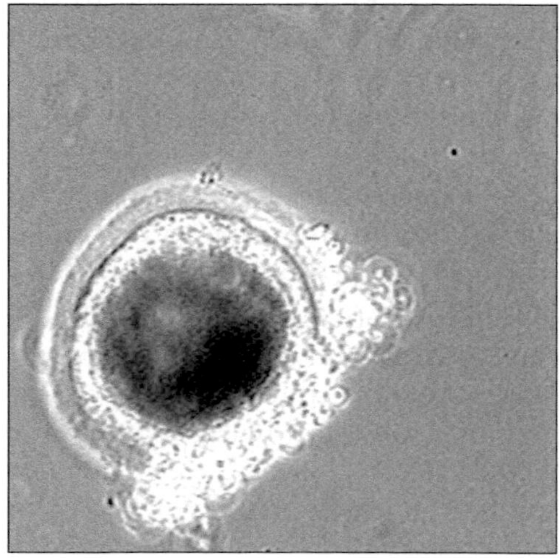

Figure 4-13
The equine oocyte with some cumulus cells still attached.

🗝 Equine oocytes, like those of other species, are ovulated as 2° oocytes, not as 1° oocytes as once believed. Once this 2° oocyte is discharged from the follicle at ovulation it is referred to as the ovum.

✓ The ovum is contained within the cumulus-oocyte complex (COC), the average size of which in the horse is around 2.5 mm (250 μ).

✓ Freshly ovulated ova can be distinguished from retained ova by the presence of a variable number of intact cumulus cells and a distinct perivitelline space in the fresh ova. The cumulus cells are shed shortly after ovulation.

🗝 Meiosis resumes when and if the ovum is penetrated by a sperm.

Fertilization

🗝 Fertilization of equine ova occurs in the ampulla of the uterine tube of the mare.

✓ Sperm transport and distribution in the uterus following insemination or ejaculation appears to have two phases:

A rapid transport phase in which some sperm are found within the uterine tube in a matter of minutes following their deposition.

A slower phase of transport involving uterine smooth muscle contractions, endometrial and oviductal cellular ciliary action, fluid currents within the uterus, and sperm flagellar action accounting for the major forces propelling sperm to the fertilization site. This slower phase delivers sperm to the fertilization site by two hours and peaks by four hours after insemination in the mare.

✓ A sperm reservoir is found in the cervical crypts of the cow, goat, and ewe. Such a reservoir in the pig is found at the uterotubal junction. In the mare, a reservoir has not been documented to occur, however, there are deep, edematous, longitudinal mucosal folds at the uterotubal junction during estrus. It has been suggested that these deep furrows may constitute the pathway to the uterine tube in the mare and act as the primary sperm storage site for the mare, similar to the sow.

✓ The uterotubal junction is thought to be the main site for capacitation and selection of sperm in the mare. Research in the mare indicates that stallion sperm is capacitated within a short period of time following its intrauterine insemination.

🗝 The diameter of the preovulatory 2° oocyte, fertilized and nonfertilized ova, and cleaving embryo is the same and does not change until formation of the blastocyst stage, which usually occurs only after embryonic entry into the uterus.

✓ It has recently been documented that the oviductal embryo produces a local stimulant (PGE_2) for contractile activity of oviductal smooth muscle, orchestrating its active transport down the oviduct to the uterine horn.

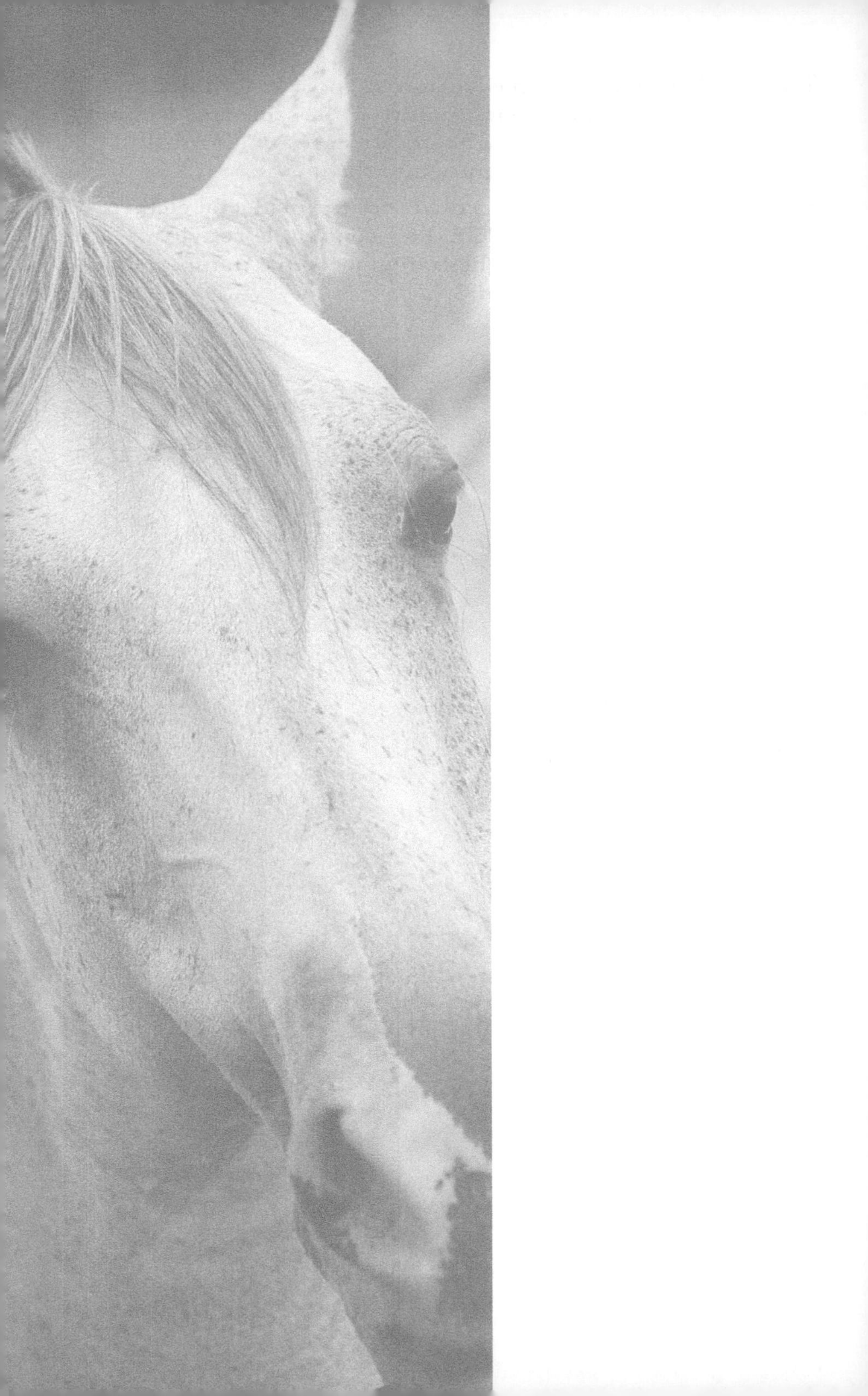

Section 5

Seasonality, the Estrous Cycle and its Manipulation and Artificial Control

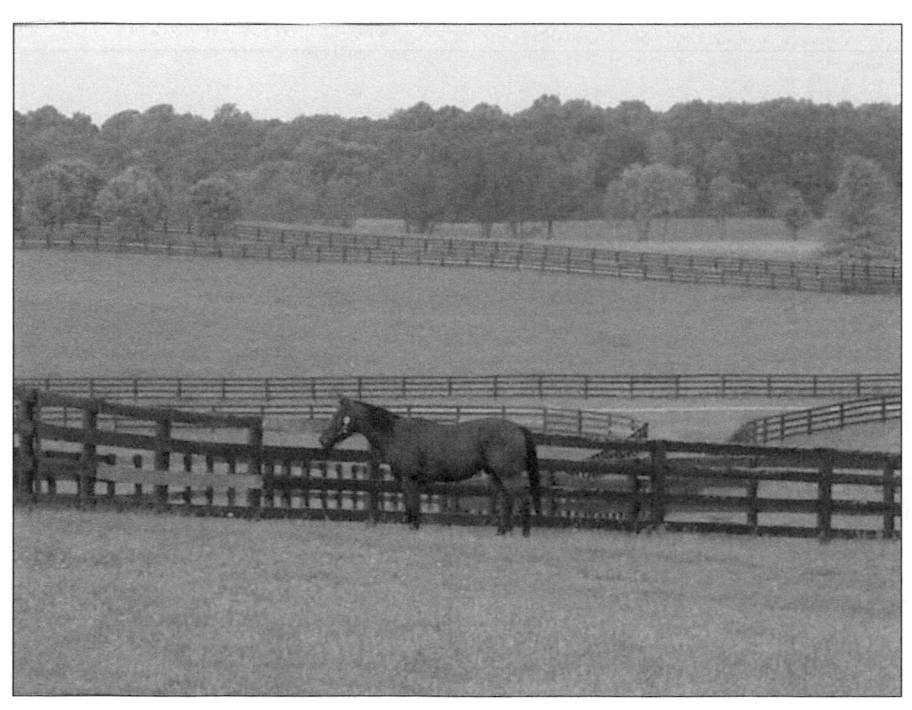

Knowing the basics of the estrous cycle, estrous induction, estrous synchronization and transitional estrous modulation is integral to success of the breeding program. It is also helpful to understand the mechanics and theory of artificial lighting programs to advance the physiologic breeding season. Becoming familiar with the physiologic and endocrine events of estrous and early pregnancy in the mare will facilitate their clinical management.

Seasonality

✓ The physiologic (natural) breeding season of the mare occurs in late spring and summer. Throughout the year, most mares will go from winter anestrus into a transitional period, into being seasonally polyestrus, into a transition period in the fall, and back into winter anestrus.

✓ During the transition from anestrus to physiologic polyestrus, the mare will frequently have variable length periods of behavioral signs of estrus without actually developing significant follicular structures or ovulating (Figure 5-1).

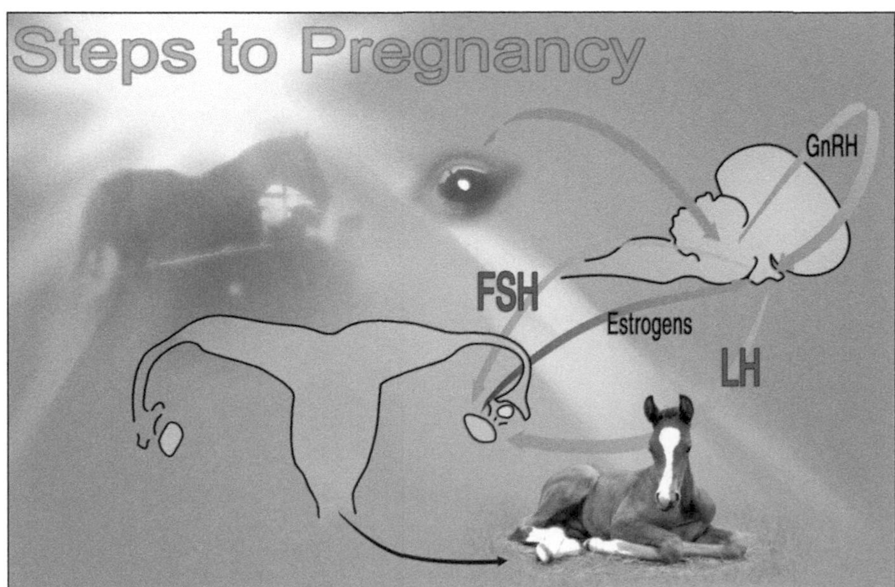

Figure 5-1 Illustration of the equine pineal-hypothalamic-pituitary-gonadal axis

✓ Daylight length (natural or induced) is the primary determinant in causing this seasonality in the temperate regions of the world. Horses nearer the equator tend to lose most if not all seasonality. Blind broodmares in the temperate regions will maintain their seasonality for one or more years after becoming completely blind.

💣 Under natural settings, periods of 15-16 hours day length (or light stimulus) act upon the pineal-hypothalamic-pituitary-gonadal axis to suppress melatonin production. Melatonin when released from the pineal gland inhibits gonadotropin (GnRH) production in the hypothalamus. Modulation of the frequency and amplitude of release of GnRH from the hypothalamus affects pituitary production and release of follicle stimulating hormone (FSH) and luteinizing hormone (LH). Ovarian receptors respond to FSH and LH inducing follicle recruitment, selection, and dominance as discussed in Section 4 (Figure 5-2).

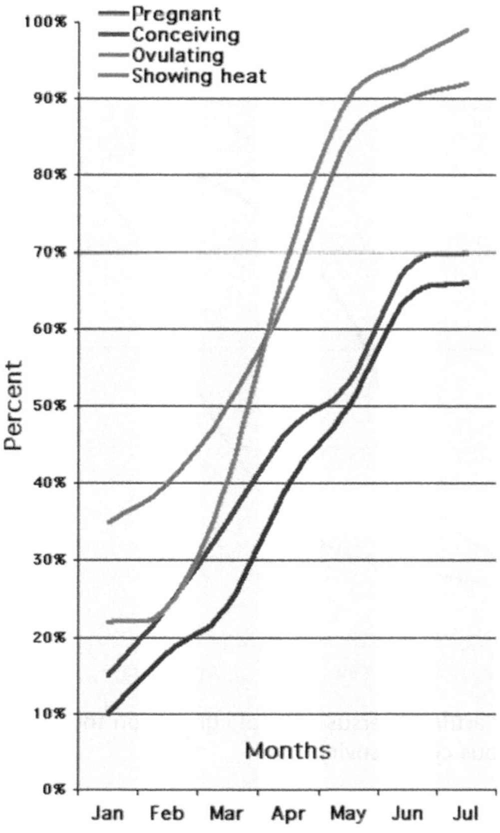

Figure 5-2 Reproductive aspects of the mare by month under natural lighting conditions in the Northern Hemisphere.

✓ Light stimulus acting on the pineal gland inhibits melatonin production and release. Therefore, the effect is a release of inhibition on the hypothalamic production and release of GnRH.

✓ The effect of artificial lighting programs on the mare can advance her entry into regular estrous cycle activity by 60-90 days when performed appropriately (Figure 5-3).

✓ To be effective the starting date should be around November 15th to December 1st in the northern temperate region.

✓ Sufficient lighting is provided by 10 ft. candles of illumination, or 107-108 lux, in a 12 x 12 ft. stall.

✓ Large groups of broodmares can be effectively managed under artificial lighting programs using floodlights in a dry lot situation provided all areas are illuminated with the minimal critical ft-candles.

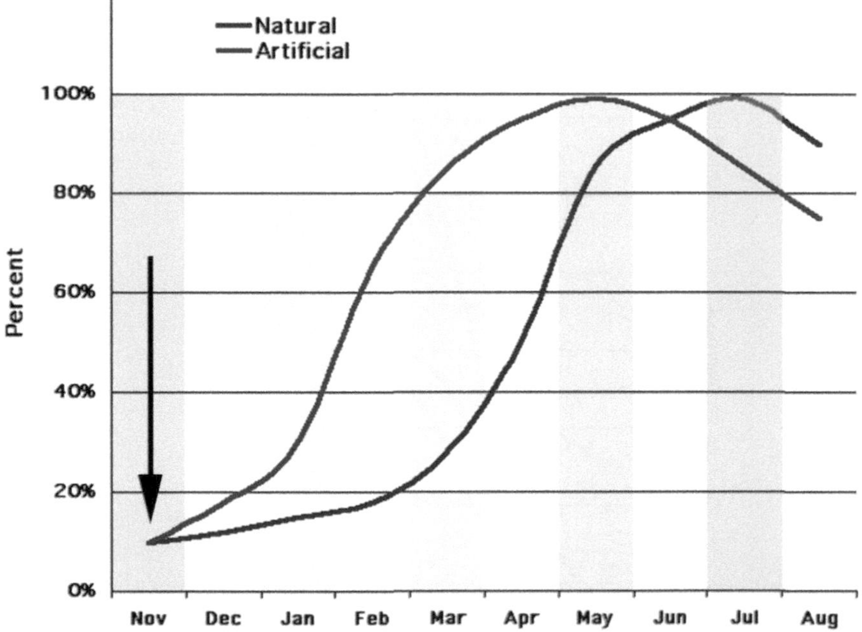

Figure 5-3 Effect of artificial versus natural lighting on the percent of mares showing regular estrous cycle activity.

The Estrous Cycle

✓ The estrous cycle is typically defined as beginning with an ovulation (day 0) and ending the day before the next ovulation. The average inter-ovulatory interval for most mares is 21 days, but the range can be from 18 to 24 days. Too short or too long may be considered an abnormality.

✓ The estrous phase (follicular phase) may last from 3 to 7 days and is dominated by one or more large (> 30 mm dia.), pre-ovulatory (Graafian) follicles, estrogen17β (E2), and behavioral signs of heat or receptivity to the stallion.

✓ P4 during estrus is typically less than 1 ng/ml in the peripheral blood.

✓ Follicular diameter at ovulation ranges from 30 to 70 mm and is most commonly around 40-45 mm.

💣 The mare ovulates 24 to 48 hours prior to the time that behavioral signs of estrus subside. This is a very important physiologic event to remember. Too many mares are bred or inseminated after they ovulate simply because they are still showing signs of heat. If the insemination or breeding occurs more than 12-14 hours after ovulation, the ovum will likely be too aged to be readily fertilizable, or if it is fertilized, will likely fail to develop into a viable embryo.

✓ During the intermediate period of 1-4 days after ovulation, E2 decreases, and before the CL begins to produce significant amounts of P4, the mare shows equivocal signs of heat or receptivity to the stallion.

💣 The diestrous phase (luteal phase) lasts 13-17 days, and is dominated by a corpus luteum (CL; or more than one corpora lutea, CLs), progesterone (P4), and behavioral signs indicating nonreceptivity to the approach of the stallion.

✓ The CL developing after an ovulation (primary CL; 1° CL) typically has a lifespan of up to 85 days. If the endometrium does not release prostaglandin-F2-alpha (PGF2) it will continue its production of progesterone and not regress.

✓ Maternal recognition of pregnancy in the mare that ovulates and is appropriately bred or inseminated is believed to be the result of the freely mobile embryo producing and secreting E2 that suppress endometrial release of PGF2. This must occur between days 12 and 14 after ovulation to be effective.

In the mare that fails to conceive, or that is not bred or exposed to a stallion, or has an early embryonic death (prior to day 12-14), the endometrium secretes PGF2 which by way of the long-loop pathway (systemic circulation) affects the CL and induces its regression (luteolysis). P4 production declines over the next 4 to 40 hours, and the mare begins to show signs of receptivity as she enters her next estrous cycle.

✓ Figure 5-4 is a schematic representation of the events of the estrous cycle of the mare.

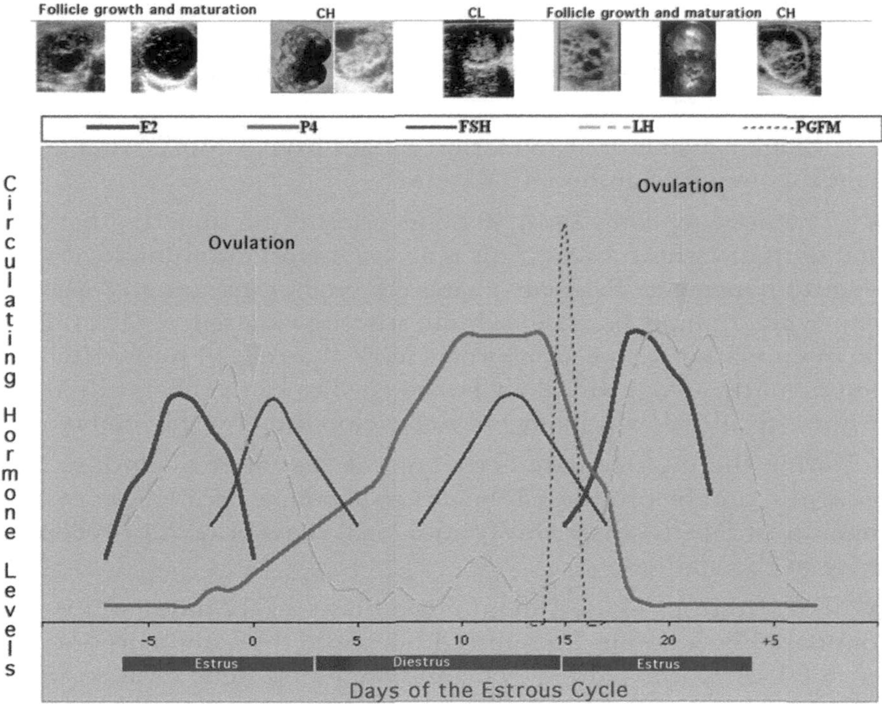

Figure 5-4 Events of the estrous cycle of the mare.

Points of Control

Progestogens (Progestin, Progesterone, P4)

✓ Available formulations include: progesterone, altrenogest, melengestrol acetate, medroxyprogesterone acetate, hydroxyprogesterone caproate, and norgestomet

✓ Use during the vernal transition (transition from winter anestrus to breeding season)

Blocks LH release from the pituitary

Blocks expression of estrous behavior

Variably inhibits follicular growth and ovulation

Effect is greater during late transition as opposed to early transition

12 to 14 day treatment periods

✓ Use to synchronize estrus

11 to 14 day treatment period

7 to 8 day treatment plus PGF2 at the end of P4 treatments

7 to 8 day treatment using (P4 +E2, P & E) plus PGF2 at the end

✓ P4 therapy alone does not inhibit follicular development in cycling mares

✓ Use to delay postpartum estrus and ovulation

Intent is to delay ovulation until after day 15 postpartum to improve conception rate by allowing more time for uterine involution.

✓ Use to suppress estrous behavior in performance mares

P4 treatments block or suppress estrous behavior to a variable extent; choice of agent depends upon cost and convenience of administration

✓ Use to assist maintenance of pregnancy

Luteal dysfunction of the 1° CL may contribute to low systemic P4 levels and may lead to early embryonic or fetal loss

Both injectable P4 and altrenogest are used to assist maintenance of pregnancy

Start of treatment can be as early as day 5 post-ovulation or beginning on the first day of a positive pregnancy diagnosis

Discontinuation of therapy: after day 100 to 150 of gestation

Monitor peripheral P4 concentration; altrenogest does not interfere with this measurement

Some pregnant mares appear to depend on an exogenous source of progestogen, especially when using altrenogest. Thus, once started, it should be continued at least through day 100 of gestation.

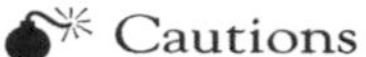
Cautions

P4 inhibits uterine polymorphonuclear leukocyte (PMN) function and diminishes uterine clearance--both important uterine defense mechanisms

Prostaglandins (PGF2-alpha and PGF2)

Considerations in the mare

Peripheral degradation is relatively slow and occurs in the lungs.

CL of the mare is not susceptible to luteolysis until day 5-6 post-ovulation.

Side-effects occur when using the natural product (dinoprost). These include sweating, diarrhea, colic, incoordination, and dragging rear limbs. These are self-limiting and most usually not life-threatening.

Analogs have less likelihood of causing these side effects.

✓ Use to terminate active CL function or induce luteolysis (80-90% efficacy)

P4 production decreases within 4h and ceases within 48h of administration

Interval to estrus and ovulation is variable and is dependent upon development of existing follicles at the time of PGF administration

In estrous synchronization programs, PGF is used on the last day of P4 treatments, or may given alone as two injections 11-14 days apart

✓ Use to terminate pregnancy or treat a pseudopregnancy

Single dose prior to day 35

Multiple daily doses (3 to 5 treatments) after day 40

✓ Use to induce ovulation

In vernal transition mares and in mares in diestrus, PGF2 induces secretion of FSH and LH

Fenprostalene given 60h after the onset of estrus induced ovulation in 81% of treated mares vs. 31% in control mares

Some practitioners believe the same effect is seen with the use of dinoprost

✓ Use to aid treatment of endometritis

PGF2 as a direct inotropic effect on myometrial contraction independent from P4 influence and aids relaxation of the cervix to promote uterine clearance.

PGF2 also mediates oxytocin release

Gonadotrophins (hCG and GnRH)

✓ Human Chorionic Gonadotrophin (hCG)

A large polypeptide hormone; half-life in the systemic circulation is 8 to 12h

Biologic activity is primarily LH-like activity in the mare

More predictable response in stimulating or advancing ovulation when used after follicles are >30-35 mm

Better response observed when used in the early part of the breeding season versus the latter

Has been shown to competitively inhibit CL growth and development when given in successive doses prior to day 39 of gestation

Antibody development occurs but cross-reactivity with endogenous LH is not clinically relevant

Two injections during the same breeding season may be the practical limit due to development of antibodies and their influence upon efficacy of hCG in inducing ovulation

✓ Gonadotropin-releasing hormone (GnRH, LHRH)

Types: native, or natural GnRH in Cystorelin™, Fertagyl™; and analogs in Factrel™ (gonadorelin HCl); Receptal™ (buserelin); Ovuplant™ (deslorelin).

Analogs can be agonists, or antagonists, and either short-, or long-acting.

To induce follicular development, hourly IV injections have been used at 2 to 20µg GnRH; alternatively, subcutaneous copolymer implants, or subcutaneous mini-pumps have been used in research settings for the same result.

Continuous high dose administration induces gonadal suppression in many species, but not the mare.

GnRH can induce LH release and thus may be able to induce ovulation as an alternative to hCG; however, this usually requires hourly injections.

Ovuplant™ implants have been shown to induce a consistent suppression of LH and FSH concentrations in systemic circulation of treated mares lasting for 10-14 days. This can cause a prolongation of the interovulatory interval. Current recommendations when using the impant for ovulation control are to remove the implant after 48 hours or administer it in the vaginal submucosa versus subcutaneously in the neck.

✓ Table 5-1 Lists the hormonal options available or approved for estrous cycle management in mares in the United States.

Options for Management

Estrous Synchronization Programs

Two PGF2 injections at 11 to 14 day intervals include hCG at 48 hours after start of estrus.

78 to 92% of treated cycling mares show estrus within 6 days and ovulate within 7-15 days after the second PGF treatment

✓ Long-term P4 (progesterone in oil or altrenogest) administration daily for 14 to 15 days usually include PGF2 on the first and last days of P4 treatment.

✓ Short-term P4 (progesterone in oil or altrenogest) administration daily for 7 to 8 days usually includes PGF2 on the last day of P4 treatment.

✓ Both P4 regimens are associated with variable days to onset of estrus (3 to 6 days) and intervals to ovulation of 8 to 15 days.

✓ P & E (150 mg P4 in oil compounded with 10 mg estradiol–17β) administered daily IM for 10 days; this usually includes PGF2 on last day of P & E treatment.

70-90% of treated cycling mares ovulated within 10 to 12 days after end of P & E

No estrous synchronization protocol is sufficiently precise so that day of ovulation can be consistently controlled.

Table 5-1
Hormonal Products Available for Use in Mares in the United States

Compound	Product Trade Name	Source	Indications	Approved*	Dosages	Comments
Progestogens	Altrenogest Regumate™	Intervet, Inc. (Hoechst)	Shorten duration of transitional season; estrus suppression; estrus synchronization; supplemental P4 during gestation	Yes	0.044 mg/kg/day orally for 10-15 days	Approved only for mares in late vernal transition
	Progesterone (P4) in oil (generic)	Various	As above	No	150-300 mg/day IM for 10-15 days	Deep IM injections; Can be combined with E2 for better suppression of follicular growth
Estrogens	Estradiol 17-β Estradiol benzoate (generic)	Various	Induction of estrus behavior in jump mares	No	10 mg/day IM	Effective only in absence of CL's or for use in winter anestrus or in ovariectomized mares; Can be combined with P4 for better suppression of follicular growth

continued

Table 5-1 continued

Compound	Product Trade Name	Source	Indications	Approved*	Dosages	Comments
GnRH (Gonadotropin-Releasing Hormone)	Gonadorelin Factrel™ Cystorelin™ Fertagyl™	——— Fort Dodge Merial Intervet, Inc.	Stimulation of follicular growth; stimulation of LH release and ovulation	No	50mcg IM or IV	Not cost effective for use in winter anestrus; not as effective as hCG in stimulation of ovulation.
	Deslorelin Ovuplant™	Fort Dodge Animal Health	For inducing ovulation within 48h in estrous mares with an ovarian follicle greater than 30 mm in diameter.	Yes	One implant containing 2.1 mg deslorelin SQ in the mare	Effective when follicle size meets minimum recommendations; removal of implant at 48h is advised; has been applied intra-vaginally.
hCG (human Chorionic Gonadotropin)	Chorionic Gonadotropin (generic)	Various	For inducing ovulation.	No	1,500 to 5,000 I.U., IM or IV	Effective for accelerating ovulation time in mares with follicle diameter > 35mm;
Follicle Stimulating Hormone	F.S.H.-P Injectable	Sioux Biochemical	Stimulation of follicular growth.	Yes	10 to 50 mg, IM, IV, or SQ	Little to no benefit in the mare.
Prostaglandin[1] (PGF2-alpha)	Dinoprost tromethamine	———	For its luteolytic effect to control	Yes	1 mg/100 lbs, or 10 mcg/kg body	Dose can be reduced to 2.5 – 5.0 mcg/kg and

continued

						retain its efficacy in luteolysis; lower doses recommended to minimize side effects which include sweating, colic, and mild ataxia.
	Alfaprostol Alfavet™	Vetem S.P.A., Milano, Italy	For inducing luteolysis as above.	Yes	6 mcg/kg of body weight, IM	Effective in luteolysis; fewer side effects observed
	Cloprostenol Estrumate™	Schering-Plough	For inducing luteolysis as above.	No	250 mcg IM	Effective in luteolysis; fewer side effects observed
	Fluprostenol Equimate™	Bayer	For inducing luteolysis as above.	Yes	0.55 mcg/kg of body weight, IM	Effective in luteolysis; fewer side effects observed
	Prostalene Synchrocept™	Fort Dodge	For inducing luteolysis as above.	Yes	5 mcg/kg of body weight, SQ	Effective in luteolysis; fewer side effects observed
	Luprostiol Equestrolin™	Intervet, Inc.	For inducing luteolysis as above.	Yes	7.5 mg, IM	As above
Oxytocin	Oxytocin (generic)	Various	Obstetrical: may be used as a myotonic to aid uterine	Yes	2.5 to 20 U.S.P. units IM, IV, or SQ	Can cause premature placental separation,

continued

Table 5-1 continued

Compound	Product Trade Name	Source	Indications	Approved*	Dosages	Comments
			content evacuation or to induce parturition. In surgery: may be used postoperatively following cesarean section to facilitate involution.			fetal hypoxia, and uterine rupture, especially when used at higher dose range. Use low dose when inducing parturition.

*From FDA Approved Animal Drug Products; Online Database System; http://dil.vetmed.vt.edu/NADA/NADA.cfm

[1]All formulations are readily absorbed through the skin and can cause abortion and/or bronchial spasms. Women of childbearing age, asthmatics, and persons with bronchial and other respiratory problems should exercise extreme caution when handling these products. Federal law restricts this drug to use by or on the order of a licensed veterinarian.

NOTE: Approval by the FDA does not imply commercial availability. Some pharmaceutical companies may have voluntarily discontinued their production for economic reasons.

Artificial Lighting

✓ Photoperiod and Melatonin

☞ Rhythms defined:

circadian (q24h)

circalunar (q29d)

circannual (q1y)

diurnal (occurring during the day)

nocturnal (during the night)

quotidian (occurring every day)

nyctohemeral (occurs during both night and day)

✓ The suprachiasmatic nucleus (SCN) of the hypothalamus sustains a stable circadian rhythm of neuronal activity. The phase of this rhythm can be reset by neural signals from other brain sites in a time-of-day dependent manner. The retinohypothalamic tract (RHT or RHP) is the pathway from the retina to the SCN. Prominent regulators include glutamate, acetylcholine, and melatonin.

✓ Pineal gland is an outgrowth of the forebrain. In man its functions are obscure, but in other vertebrates it acts as an endocrine gland secreting the hormone melatonin. Melatonin is secreted primarily during the night (dark hours). Light stimulus via the RHT inhibits melatonin synthesis and release.

✓ Melatonin

Tryptophan – Serotonin – Melatonin

Melatonin, secreted from the pineal during the night, is involved in the regulation of circadian rhythms. Melatonin affects the neural and metabolic activity of SCN neurons directly by high-affinity melatonin receptors located within SCN.

Melatonin indirectly inhibits gonadal function through its target tissue in the SCN

Its effective action is antagonistic to GnRH production and release from the hypothalamus.

In sheep administration of melatonin prior to the onset of the natural breeding season (short days of the Fall) advances their reproductive activity

Pharmacologic versus physiologic doses have different effects

Melatonin antagonists would be useful to alter winter anestrous in the mare; the most useful antagonist to melatonin is the influence of artificial lights

✓ Artificial lights

Intensity: 100 watt incandescent bulb in 12 ft. x 12 ft. stall; [10 ft.-candles or 107-108 lux]. The light meter of a well–equipped single lens reflex 35mm camera can be used for measurement: DIN setting (ASA) to 400, shutter speed to 0.25 sec, a light diffuser over the lens, the aperture reading should be ≥ f4; if it is then the light intensity is 10 ft.- candles, or 108 lux.

A common recommendation is to have the mare confined to a space where she is never further than 7-8 feet from a 200 watt incandescent light bulb.

Mares should be provided at least 14.5h of light (daytime plus artificial) per day, added at the end of the day not at the start of the day.

Initiation by December 1st will have mares cycling in February and starting by November 15th will have mares cycling in January.

Sources of artificial light can be from fluorescent, incandescent, or mercury vapor lamps.

Whether mares are housed indoors versus outdoors depends upon providing an equal amount of light distribution to all areas of the confinement space so that all animals under treatment have an equivalent exposure.

"Traditional" programs for artificial lighting are the lengthened day program as described above.

"Pulse lighting" or the "French method" involves a 1h duration pulse of light at 9.5 to 10.5h after the onset of darkness. A timer can be set to turn the lights on at this time each night and turn off after the 1h period. This conserves power consumption in larger facilities.

Estrus Suppression in Show and Performance Mares

✓ Little specific research has been performed in this area, but veterinarians are frequently asked by owners or trainers how to keep their mare out of estrus during shows or other performance activities.

✓ Options include long-term or strategic use of P4 supplementation using altrenogest, progesterone in oil, P4-containing implants, ovulation induction with hCG followed by P4 supplementation, long-term P+E supplementation, and placement of an indwelling intrauterine device to prolong the luteal phase of diestrus.

💣 None of the available options are consistently effective nor are they well documented in the scientific literature.

✓ Progestagens do not inhibit follicular development, therefore mares will continue to ovulate during attempted estrus suppression treatment periods. Many mares will fail to have behavioral signs of estrus suppressed.

✓ Use of a 30-35 mm glass ball or marble as an intrauterine device to extend the luteal phase has been studied. Five of 12 mares (42%) receiving the sterile glass ball intrauterine implants had a prolonged luteal phase lasting for up to 88 days following placement. This may be an option to consider for many owners wishing to have a non-hormonal therapy applied with apparently minimal long-term effect on the future breeding potential of their mare.

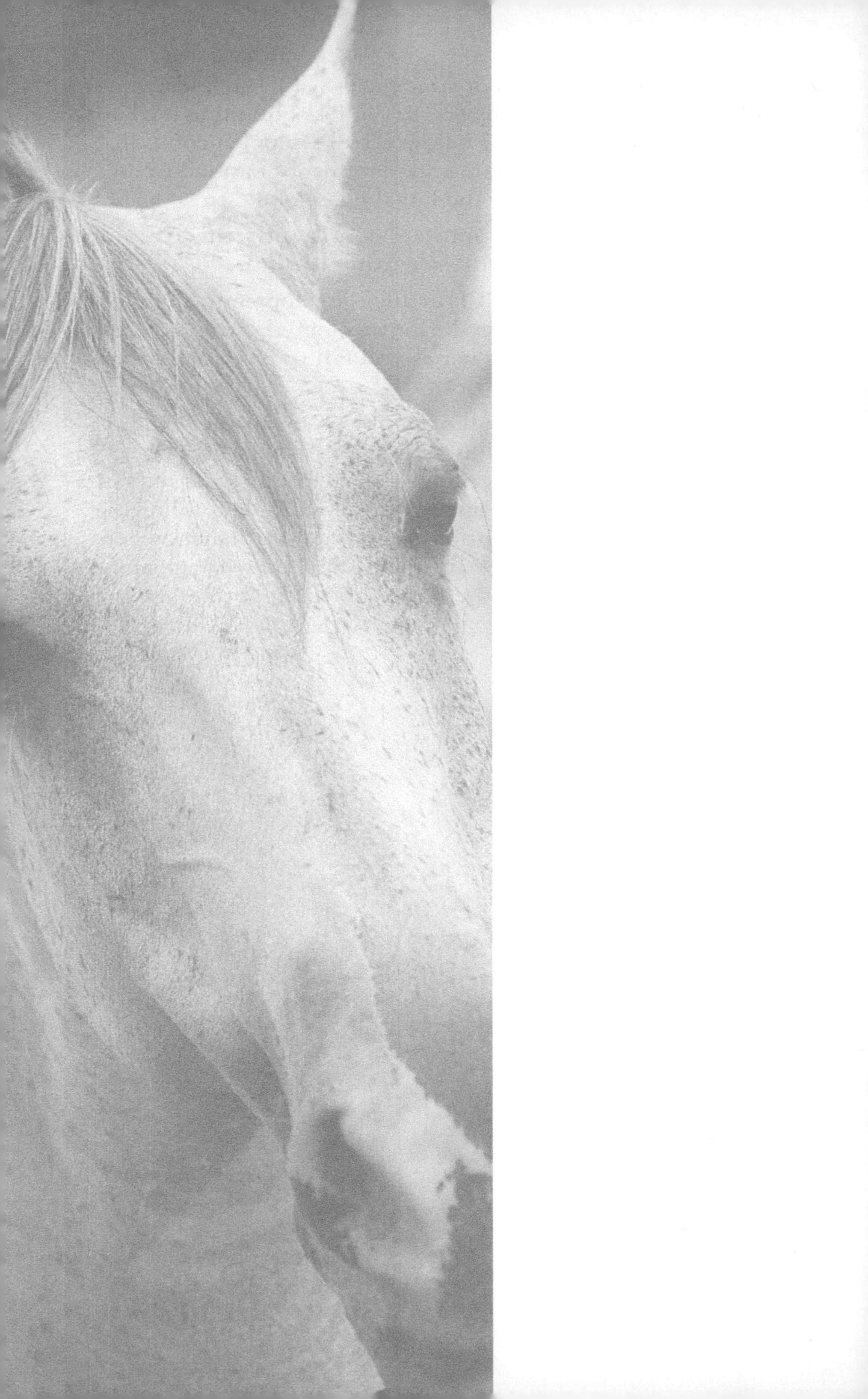

Section 6
Breeding Serviceability Exam of the Mare

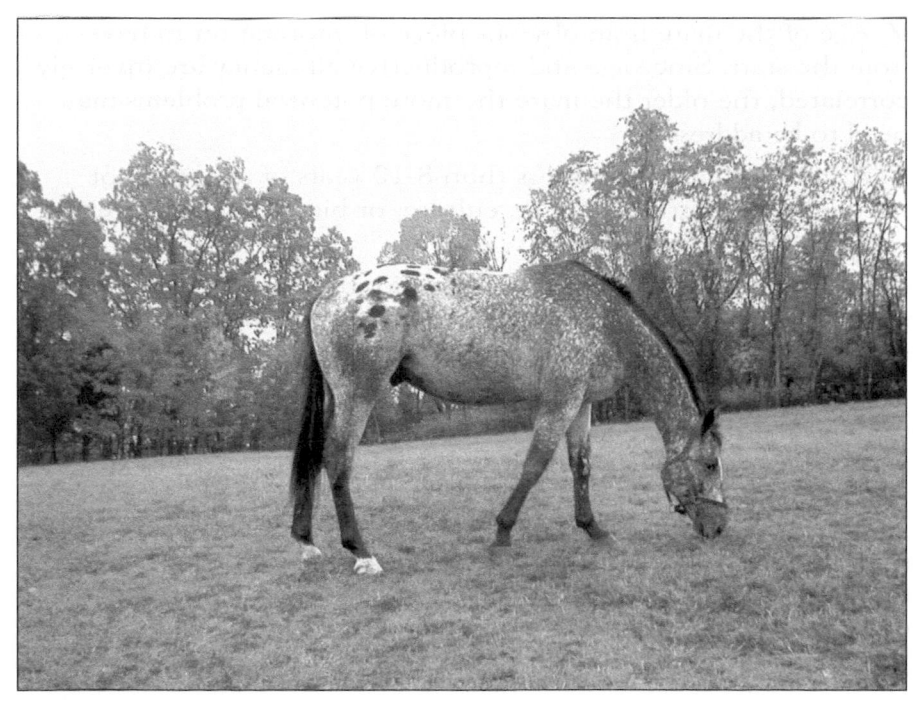

Mares are examined for health and breeding ability at the beginning of each new season, prior to sale or purchase, and when they are perceived to have a problem conceiving or maintaining pregnancy. In Section 1 I discussed my reasoning for choosing to call this a breeding serviceability exam rather than by its more common term, the breeding soundness exam.

History and Signalment

✓ Determining the reason(s) behind the client's request for the exam will help determine how in depth your diagnostics may need to be. Determining how the client perceives the problem will help focus your efforts.

✓ Indications for breeding serviceability examination include:

> Repeat breeders, barren mares, prepurchase examinations, habitual aborters, vaginal discharge, urine poolers, cervical lacerations, rectovaginal tears and fistulas (prior to surgical repair), suspected luteal insufficiency, irregular cycles, physiologic anestrus, chronic uterine infection, pyometra, hydometra, mucometra, multiple endometrial cysts, palpable uterine abnormalities (neoplasia), and mares over 12 years of age who have not had a foal within the last year.

✓ Age of the mare is an obvious piece of information to have from the start. Since age and reproductive efficiency are inversely correlated, the older the mare the more potential problems may need to be addressed.

✓ A maiden mare that is less than 8-10 years of age may not need an endometrial cytology, culture, or biopsy unless a prepurchase exam is involved.

✓ A barren mare that returns to estrus for the third time in a given season in spite of being inseminated appropriately to an otherwise proven stallion will need significantly more intense scrutiny.

☞ Some typical questions to ask: Was the mare having regular estrous cycles? How long was her last estrus? How long did she go between cycles? Was she ovulating? How was this determined? How were her signs of estrus determined? Was she teased with a stallion? How was her readiness for breeding determined? If bred, was the stallion proven? If the stallion was proven, was the mare examined early after ovulation (day 1-3) for evidence of post-breeding endometritis? Was there any evidence of a purulent discharge from her vulva? Have you noticed matted debris on her tail? Did she return to estrus too soon after her last ovulation or cycle? Did she conceive and have an early embryonic death? Did she conceive twins? Was she pregnant at or around 45 days? When was her last foal delivered? Was the last foaling normal or was there a problem at delivery? Was the foal healthy at birth? Did the foal survive to weaning or beyond?

✋ Additional questions to consider: How was she bred or inseminated and by whom? Was the semen evaluated? If so, how and by whom? Is she the only mare on your farm being bred? Was she at a breeding farm? If so, are other mares at the same farm, or being bred to the same stallion, having problems too?

✓ The goal is not only to find out as much information as possible about the mare, but also attempt to begin to define the problem from the start.

✓ Was there a problem in teasing and recognition of estrus? This may indicate a management or behavior problem.

✓ Was the mare bred at the appropriate time to optimize her chance to conceive? This may indicate a management problem.

✓ Did she fail to conceive and return to estrus? This may indicate a problem intrinsic to the mare or a problem with the stallion or his semen.

✓ Did she conceive and lose her pregnancy? This may indicate a problem intrinsic to the mare (age, uterine environment) more so than with the stallion, but he cannot be entirely eliminated from the problem as yet.

✓ Did she lose her pregnancy after day 45? This may indicate a problem intrinsic to the mare (age, uterine environment). The stallion may be exonerated here.

✓ The BSE can be performed during any stage of the estrous cycle but it is easiest during estrus when the cervix is relaxed and immune defenses highest. Should any contamination of the uterus occur due to the techniques, the mare is more able to clear the contaminants.

Physical Examination

✋ The primary reason you may be asked to examine a mare may be for a reproductive problem, but do not overlook the fact that systemic problems may potentially influence reproductive efficiency.

✓ Body condition is directly related to reproductive efficiency (refer to Section 3, Nutrition)

✓ The mare should have suitable conformation and acceptable feet and lower limbs to be able to support the added stress and weight of advanced gestation.

If examining the mare for prepurchase, the physical exam should take primary importance before proceeding with the reproductive aspects.

✓ Common laboratory tests (CBC, serum chemistry, urinalysis, fecal egg count, and EIA and or EAV serology) may be individually selected depending upon the mare's history and/or your findings on the physical exam.

✓ Eyes, teeth, heart, lungs, and digestive tract form and function must all receive at least a cursory examination.

✓ Mammary gland size and symmetry should be examined even though it may not be possible to assess its function at the time of your exam.

✓ Symptoms of equine Cushing's Disease or peripheral Cushing-like syndrome should be investigated further (see Section 11). These may include laminitic rings on the hooves, hirsutism, loss of muscle mass, increased tendency for sweating or 'salty' hair coat, and increased susceptibility to infections (parasitism, pneumonia, subsolar abscesses).

Three physical barriers exist between the environment and the endometrium: the vulva, the vestibulo-vaginal sphincter, and the cervix. During parturition, natural service, artificial insemination, or examination of the reproductive tract, microorganisms may invade or be introduced into the endometrial space. These are usually engulfed by leukocyte phagocytosis or eliminated mechanically by uterine clearance. However, due to a variety of anatomic or physiologic function abnormalities ("wind sucking" or poor perineal conformation, decreased uterine clearance, etc.) both pathogenic and nonpathogenic microorganisms can initiate an inflammatory event that overrides the normal uterine immune response.

External Perineum

✓ See Section 4 for a discussion on perineal anatomy.

✓ The tail should be examined for evidence of debris collected from vulvar discharge.

✓ The relationship of the vulva to the anal sphincter should be noted. The slope of the vulva with respect to perpendicular should be observed, along with the relationship of the dorsal commissure of the vulva to the ischial floor. These two variables can be measured and used in a calculation defined as Pascoe's Caslick Index. The effective length (L) is the distance from the dorsal commissure of the vulva to the ischial floor. The angle of declination is the difference in the measured angle of the vulva from vertical (A). The product of A and L is Pascoe's Caslick Index. This index can then serve as a tool to help the practitioner determine the need for Caslick's surgery or vulvoplasty (Figure 6-1). ⊙

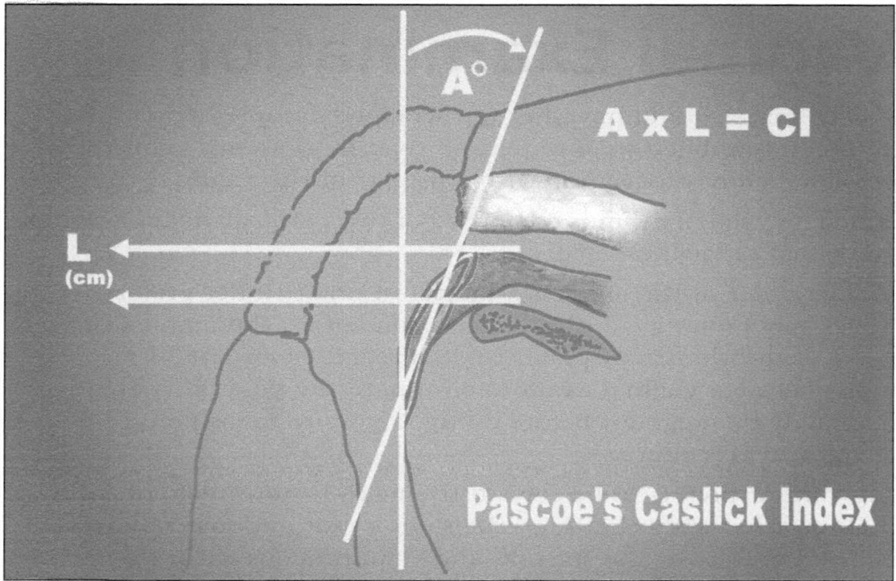

Figure 6-1 Observations to be made when examining the perineum of the mare and their use in calculating Pascoe's Caslick's Index.

✓ Pascoe's Caslick Index: Mares with a value < 100 are within normal limits; mares with a value > 150 will benefit from the surgery; mares with values between 100-150 are questionable.

✓ Before any washing or scrubbing occurs for the more invasive internal exam, the clitoris and clitoral sinus should be swabbed with a sterile culturette to collect a sample for bacterial culture and isolation of *Taylorella equigenitalis* (CEMO), *Pseudomonas aeruginosa*, and *Klebsiella pneumoniae*. These are the most common bacteria transmitted venereally.

✓ Special culture requirements exist for CEMO. Contact your state veterinary diagnostic laboratory for their recommendations.

✓ Another technique to evaluate the effective closure of the vulva is to part the lips slowly from side-to-side to expose the pink mucous membranes just inside. No less than 1 inch on either side should be exposed before the mucous membrane apposition on each side is broken and an air gap is created.

✓ Defects in the vulvar lips, anal sphincter, or perineal body should be noted and their effect on compromising this first line of anatomical or physical barrier of defense against uterine infection should be assessed.

Vaginal Examination

✓ The mare should have her tail wrapped completely and the perineum scrubbed with water and soap in as aseptic manner as possible before proceeding with this part of the exam.

🗝 The vaginal exam is comprised of two parts: manual or digital, and visual or vaginoscopic.

✓ The order of the exam is a matter of practitioner preference. Some may prefer to do the visual exam before the manual or vice versa. Still others may prefer to do a rectal exam and ultrasonography before a vaginal exam to eliminate the possibility that the mare may be pregnant before doing any more invasive type of diagnostic procedure.

The author prefers to be certain the mare is not pregnant first, then proceed with obtaining the samples for endometrial cytology and culture at the start of, and simultaneous with, the manual vaginal exam. This minimizes the chance of contaminating the sample to be obtained for possible bacterial culture with contaminants from the more distal reproductive tract. ⊙ See CD for Ultrasound of Barren Mare (Video 6-1)

✓ The manual exam is performed in an aseptic manner using a sterile obstetrical glove or sleeve and sterile obstetrical lubricant. The goal is to feel the internal limits of the vagina, the area of the vestibule, the vestibulovaginal sphincter, the anterior vaginal fornix, the external os of the cervix, and the lumen of the cervix in their entirety.

💣 Palpable defects involving the cervix must be noted and considered serious detriments to the breeding serviceability of the mare.

✓ The vaginoscopic exam is performed again in an aseptic manner using a sterile disposable cardboard or plastic speculum or a sterile stainless steel Thoroughbred-type vaginal speculum lubricated with a minimal amount of sterile obstetrical lube (Figure 6-2). ⊙

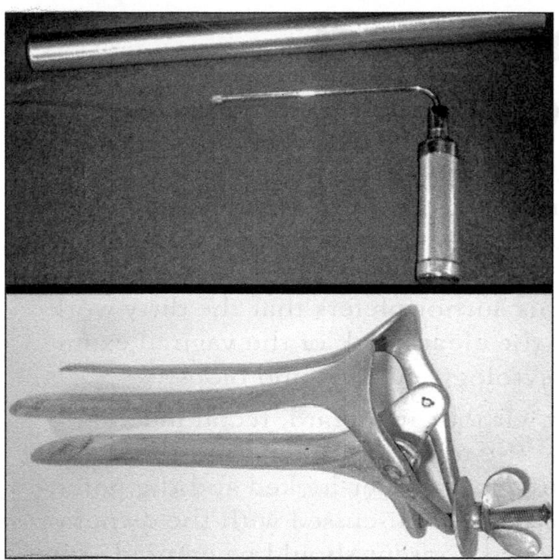

Figure 6-2 Speculums used in the vaginoscopic examination.
Top; a disposable cardboard type. Bottom; a stainless steel Thoroughbred type.

🗝 The vaginal mucous membrane should be light pink at initial observation and will blanch to pale pink with time of observation. The underlying vascularity will become more prominent as the exam proceeds.

🗝 In estrus, the mucous membrane will be moist pink. In diestrus and during pregnancy, the mucous membrane surface will be comparatively pale and dry.

✓ The external os of the cervix in diestrus will be suspended in the anterior fornix and appear to be tightly closed. This change is even more dramatic during early pregnancy. In estrus, the external os has a glistening, moist, or edematous appearance and is pink; it lays on the floor of the anterior vagina. In anestrus, the external os is both pale and dry and may be very lax or loose; the observer may be able to look directly into the uterine body through the cervical lumen.

🗝 Types of cervical discharge to be noted are purulent, mucopurulent, mucoid, and hemorrhagic. Samples for culture and cytology should be obtained upon their first observation, if they have not already been obtained previously at a manual exam.

⦿ Whenever sampling for bacterial culture and identification is intended as part of the diagnostic procedure, use of a sterile nonbacteriostatic nonbactericidal obstetrical lubricant is recommended. See CD for list of suppliers.

Rectal Exam and Ultrasonography

🗝 As mentioned above, performing the diagnostics of the breeding serviceability exam are a matter of practitioner preference. The rectal exam and ultrasonography almost always go hand-in-hand. Whether they precede the vaginal exam or follow it, is a matter of choice. This author prefers that the dirty work of the rectal exam precede the clean work of the vaginal exam and obtaining samples for cytology, culture, and biopsy.

💣 The rectal exam is not without its hazard, rectal mucosal perforation or tearing being the most serious and life-threatening to the mare. This point must not be over-looked and the potential for damage to the mare must be discussed with the owner or responsible agent. An informed consent should be granted either verbally or in writing before proceeding. The concern for rectal tearing is greatest in young mares, fractious mares, mares of lighter breeding such as Arabian, and in pony mares.

💣 Remember rings, wrist jewelry, and watches should be removed!

💣 Fingernails must be clipped short!

💣 Restraint of the mare is a serious concern, not only with respect to the possibility of inducing a rectal tear, but also with respect to the examiner's continued health and well-being. Stocks are preferred. When not available, the mare's rear can be positioned just through the door of a stall, where the door jam can serve as a modicum of protection from potential kicking attempts by the mare. Application of a nose twitch or shoulder twitch by the handler at the mare's head may be helpful. Sedation may also be necessary in some mares, but never rely on sedation as a security protection. Sedated mares may still kick!

✓ The examiner wearing a full length obstetrical sleeve, well lubricated with mineral oil or obstetrical lubricant, should advance the hand into and through the anal sphincter and carefully remove all fecal material from the rectum and small colon as far forward as is possible to reach.

✓ The limits of the bony pelvis should be felt and any limitations that may exist to prevent delivery per vaginum of a normal foal should be noted.

✓ The cervix should be identified, its external os and anterior limit defined to assess its length. The cervical lumen should be compressed from dorsal to ventral to determine how flaccid it may be and its width and tubularity noted.

✓ A mare in estrus will have a relatively short and flaccid cervix, easily flattened, and each of 3 to 4 fingers of the examiner's hand may be placed between its lateral limits.

✓ A diestrous cervix is much more tubular, less flaccid, and comparatively longer.

✓ A pregnant mare's cervix is very tubular, narrow, and elongated.

⊙ The horns and body of the uterus can be palpated by reaching forward with the hand, fingers held together and extended. At the near maximal reach of the examiner, the hand and fingers are gently and carefully directed down and the fingers and palm cupped towards the pubis and the arm retracted as a sweeping motion is initiated. This will usually result in trapping the uterus within the confines of the examiner's hand as it becomes restricted by the broad ligaments (Figure 6-3). See CD for demonstration of laparoscopy exam of the reproductive tract (Video 6-2).

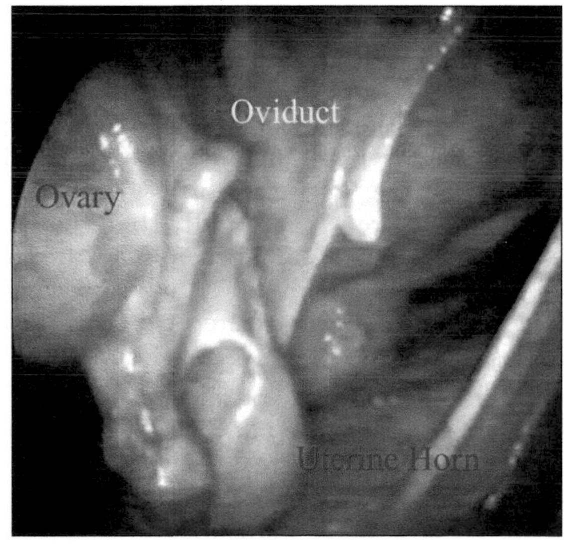

Figure 6-3
Laparoscopic view of the mare's ovary, oviduct, and tip of the uterine horn.

✓ Sweeping up the left and right horns and across the uterine body, the examiner should note uterine horn size and symmetry, the presence of any fluid within the uterus, and areas of increased or decreased tone indicating possible pathology (uterine cyst).

✓ Focal enlargement in one horn with fluid and decreased tone may indicate pregnancy.

✓ The ovary can be palpated by keeping the uterine horn in hand, sweeping to its anteriolateral extremity or tip, and then reaching approximately a hand-width anterior and lateral. The firm mass of the ovary will usually be detected. It should be cupped in the palm of the hand and its four surfaces examined with the fingertips.

✓ Follicles usually protrude above the ovarian surface and have a fluid fluctuance. Their greatest diameter, tone, and location on the ovary should be recorded.

🔑 CLs within the ovary of the mare are not identifiable on most rectal examinations.

✓ Both ovaries are examined for size, symmetry, position in the abdominal cavity, and follicular activity with respect to the time of the year.

✓ Mares in estrus should have at least one follicle present that is at least 30-35 mm in diameter on one or both ovaries.

✓ Mares in diestrus may have one or more small follicles palpable, and may even have a pre-ovulatory (mid-diestrus) follicle palpable (i.e., > 35 mm). Determining the presence of a CL on the ovary of a mare at any time of her cycle is usually not possible by palpation.

✓ A mare that has just ovulated, may have a palpable depression where the follicle was present. As the corpus hemorrhagicum (CH) develops, this area may have a crackling or crinkling feel as the examiner disrupts fibrin within the collapsed and hemorrhagic structure. Occasionally there may be increased sensitivity by the mare when palpating a CH. She may grunt, groan, wince, or kick as it is examined. Usually, by day 5, the structure of the CH blends into the texture of the ovarian parenchyma and is not as easily identified.

🔑 Ultrasonography of the reproductive tract is no longer a specialized procedure but an expected standard of practice. A low profile 5.0 MHz transrectal ultrasound linear transducer is most commonly used for this exam, but some practitioners may choose the 7.5 MHz linear transducer for better resolution or detail. The 3.0 MHz transducer, while still in use by some, provides too little fine detail to be of significant benefit.

⊙ Ultrasonography should follow the rectal exam since the rectum and small colon are already cleared of fecal material, and the examiner is already familiar with the location of the internal structures to be visualized. See CD for demonstration of ultrasound examinations of an anestrous mare (Video 6-1). Additional ultrasound exams are found in Videos 6-5, 6-6, and 6-7.

✓ The sequence of the exam does not matter as long as the examiner is consistent in his or her pattern of exam and that both ovaries, both uterine horns, uterine body, and the cervix in its entirety are evaluated.

✓ The ovaries are examined for overall size and specifically for follicle size and location, presence or absence of CLs or CHs. Each structure identified should be recorded or documented by videotape or static image capture (Figures 6-4, 6-5, and 6-6). ⊙

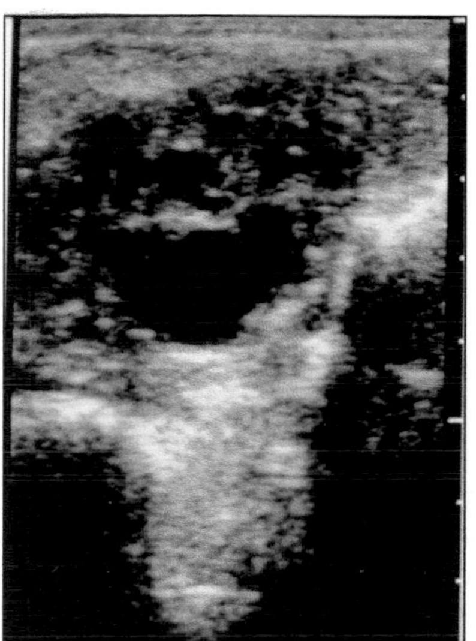

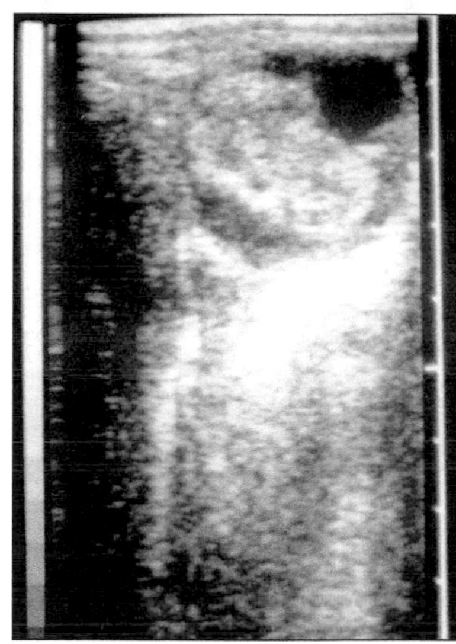

Figure 6-4 (Left) Ultrasonogram of the mare's ovary showing follicles.

Figure 6-5 (Right) Ultrasonogram of the mare's ovary showing a corpus luteum (CL).

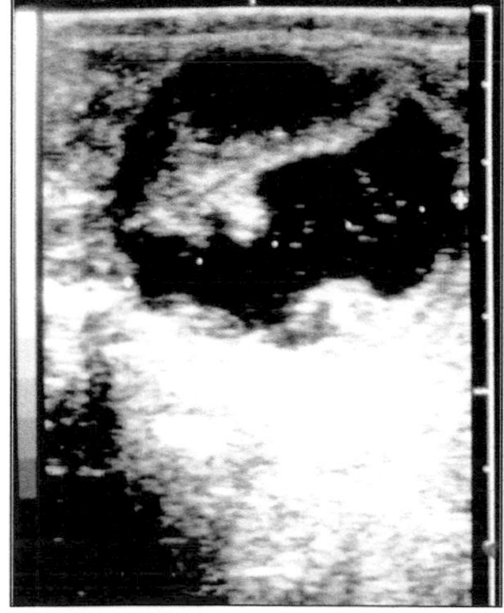

Figure 6-6 Ultrasonogram of the mare's ovary showing a corpus hemorrhagicum (CH).

✓ The uterus (both horns and body) should be examined for fluid (hypoechoic or black areas) within the lumen, endometrial cysts, foreign bodies, pregnancy, and character of endometrial fold architecture (Figures 6-7, 6-8, 6-9, 6-10, and 6-11). ⊙

⊙ See CD for demonstration for US exams of mares with uterine fluid (Video 6-3).

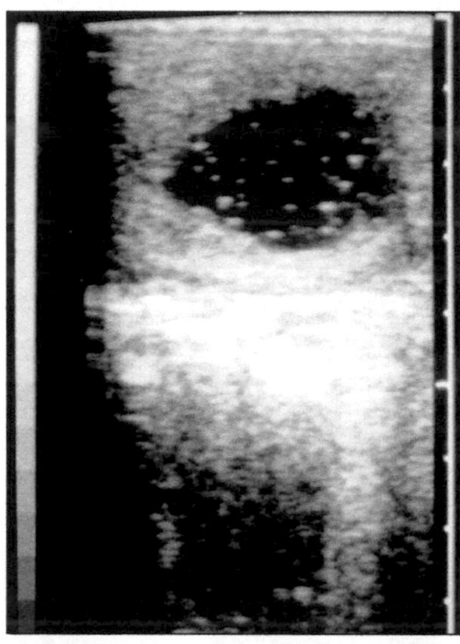

Figure 6-7 Ultrasonogram of the mare's uterine horn in cross-section showing a large accumulation of hypoechoic fluid in the uterine lumen. This mare had urometra.

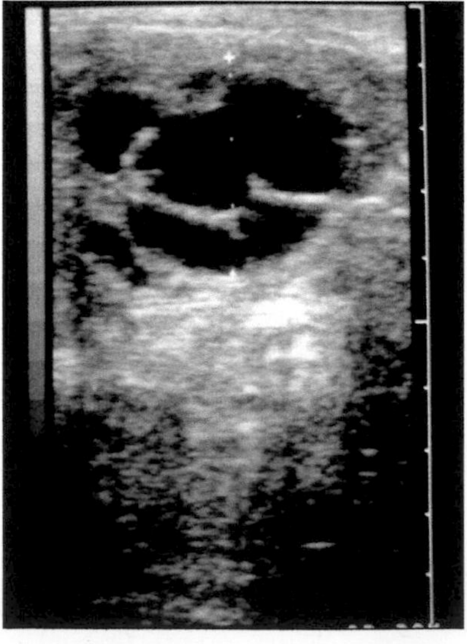

Figure 6-8 Ultrasonogram of the mare's uterine horn in cross-section showing a large endometrial cyst.

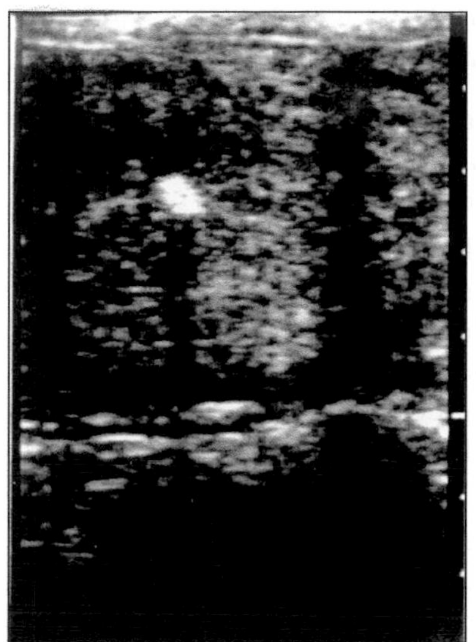

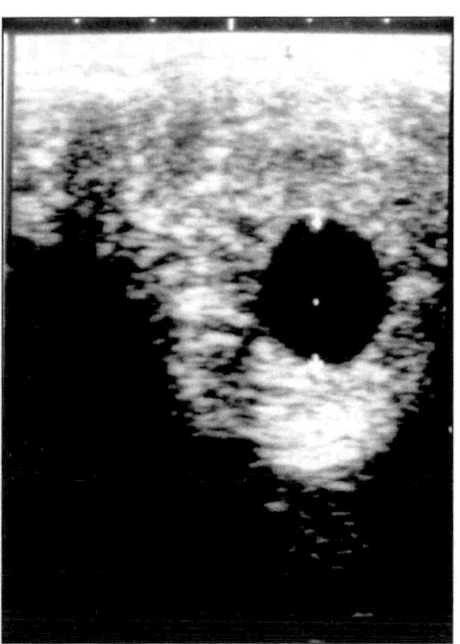

Figure 6-9 (Left) Ultrasonogram of the mare's uterine horn in cross-section showing a foreign body within the uterine lumen. Note the object is hyperechoic and has a shadowing effect cast below it. This was the cotton tip of an endometrail culturette inadvertently left in the mare during a procedure for endometrial cytology and culture.

Figure 6-10 (Right) Ultrasonogram of a mare's uterine horn in cross-section showing a 15 day embryonic vesicle.

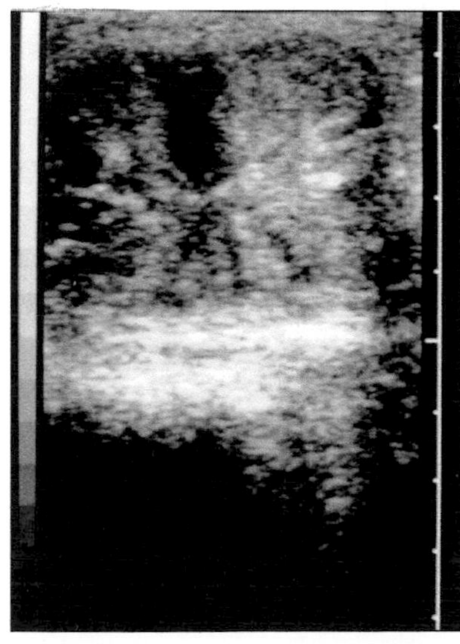

Figure 6-11 Ultrasonogram of a mare's uterine horn in cross-section revealing endometrial folds that are hypoechoic. This sign is consistent with endometrial edema of estrus.

Endometrial Cytology

✓ The technique for obtaining the samples for endometrial cytology and culture are very similar and can sometimes be accomplished using the same instrument or culturette.

✓ The mare is restrained as per rectal exam with the tail wrapped and her perineum scrubbed as per the vaginal exam. Remember you do not want to introduce any contaminants into her more cranial reproductive tract as part of your diagnostics, and you are not interested in sampling contaminants from her more caudal tract. Use as sterile a technique as can be accomplished in your given surroundings.

✓ The practitioner is gloved with a sterile obstetrical sleeve and has non-bacteristatic lubricant applied. With the sterile hand the opened end of the sterile endometrial culturette is grasped and palmed to protect it during introduction through the vulva and vagina (Figure 6-12). The index finger, or index and middle fingers, are gently introduced into the external os of the cervix and manipulated through the entire length of the cervical lumen. The culturette is then passed next to the one or between the two guide fingers. The swab of the culturette is exposed to the endometrial surface and held stationary for several seconds to absorb fluid. Moving or 'swabbing' the tip is discouraged as the tip of many swabs may dislodge or break off with too much manipulation.

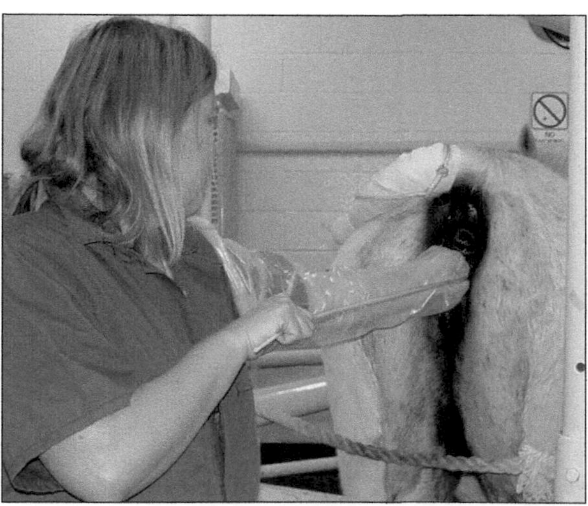

Figure 6-12 The procedure for obtaining samples for endometrial cytology and culture can be performed simultaneously and should be accomplished in an aseptic manner.

✓ Many different endometrial culturettes are commercially available with advantages and disadvantages to each. The basics you should look for are:

Double-guarded to protect the swab from distal tract contamination,

Tightly adherent calcium alginate swab that does not dislodge,

Flexible tip holding the swab, enough to bend 90° without breaking off,

A design acceptable to you as the user of the product that will allow you to obtain both culture and cytology samples with one entry into the cervix/uterus.

✓ The author prefers to use a single endometrial swab and make a smear from the tip of this swab onto a sterile glass slide prior to introducing the same tip into the transport culture media for sending the sample to the lab or bacterial culture and sensitivity (Figure 6-13). ⊙

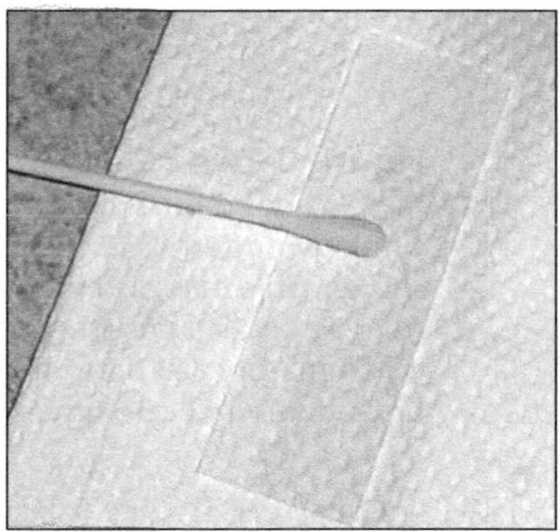

Figure 6-13
Making a smear for endometrial cytology onto a sterile glass slide prior to introducing the swab tip into the transport culture media is a simple and effective method for accomplishing both procedures with one technique and one instrument.

✓ One or two new microscope slides can be enclosed in small mailer packets (cardboard or plastic) and gas or steam sterilized. This protects them in storage and transport to and from farms, and prevents them from breakage. They can additionally be sealed in a plastic or paper outer wrapping to safeguard their sterility until opened for use.

⊙ The microscope slide is allowed to air dry and then stained using the Dif-Quick™ stain before evaluation under low (200x), high (400x), and oil immersion (1,000x). A second slide may also be prepared and set aside for gram stain if desired by the practitioner (Figure 6-13B on CD).

✓ The goal of the endometrial cytology exam is to screen the mare for evidence of inflammatory cells within the uterine lumen. It provides little to no benefit in staging of the estrous cycle. This is intended to be a "stall side" or "on the farm" test where the result can be determined within minutes of sampling, and an opinion can be expressed as to the health of the mare's uterine environment.

✓ An inflammatory pattern found on endometrial cytology has a positive and direct correlation with isolation of pathogenic bacteria from endometrial culture samples obtained at the same time in the same mare. If inflammation is evident, the culture should be submitted to an appropriate laboratory.

✓ There are almost no polymorphonuclear leukocytes (PMNs) present in endometrial cytology samples from normal mares (Figure 6-14). ⊙

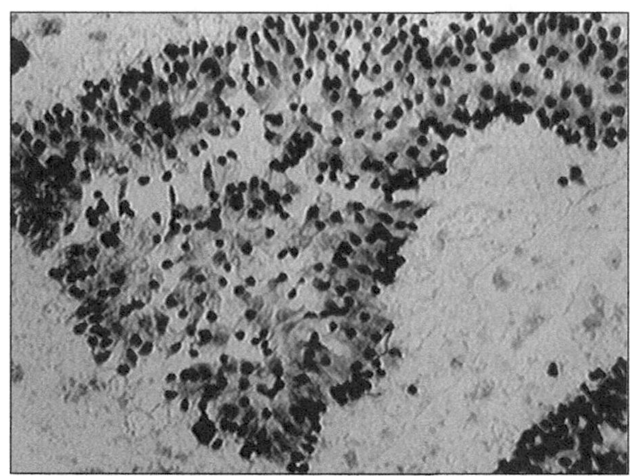

Figure 6-14 A normal mare's endometrial cytology pattern is shown. This may also be referred to as a negative inflammatory cell pattern on endometrial cytology.

✓ A positive endometrial cytology is one that has more than 1-3PMNs per 5 high power fields (Figure 6-15) ⊙. Such an inflammatory pattern supports the clinical significance of isolation and growth of pathogenic bacteria from the uterus on culture. If no bacteria were identified from a culture taken at the same time from the same mare, the practitioner should question one of three scenarios:

The bacteria died in transport to the laboratory.

The laboratory did not perform adequate testing to isolate the bacteria present.

The mare was already in a resolution phase of the infection, and all bacteria that had been present were then cleared by her cellular and non-cellular uterine defense mechanisms.

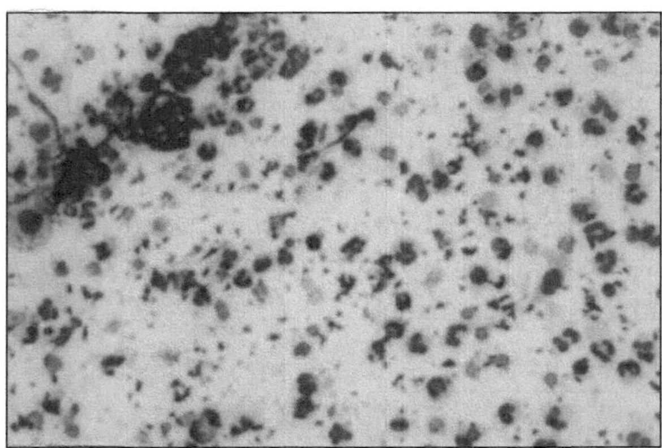

Figure 6-15 A mare's endometrial cytology pattern is shown that is inflammatory or positive. There are numerous PMNs throughout almost all high power fields (400x).

✓ If bacteria are grown and identified from an endometrial culture in the absence of an inflammatory cell pattern on endometrial cytology, their significance to the mare's reproductive health and well-being should be highly suspect.

In my experience, *Pseudomonas aeruginosa* has been identified on endometrial culture in the absence of a prominent inflammatory cell pattern on cytology. This may be the only exception.

✓ When present in the uterine environment, yeast and vegetative fungi are easily observed on endometrial cytologic samples (Figure 6-16). ⊙

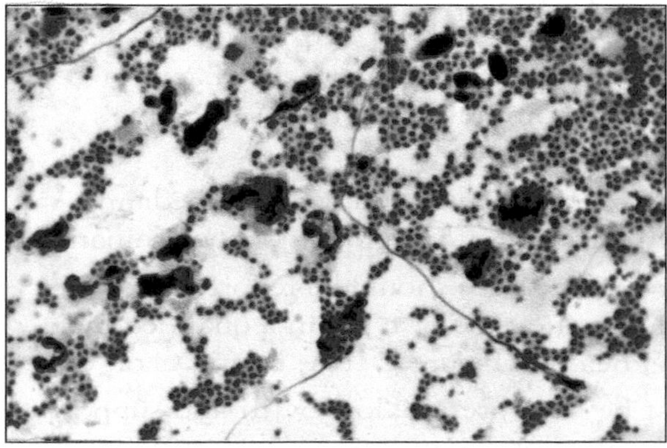

Figure 6-16 A mare's endometrial cytology on which yeast have been identified Saccharomyces spp. (400x).

✓ Cytologic examination of the uterine content may reveal patterns of chronic and acute inflammation. Plasmacytes, small mononuclear lymphocytes, macrophages, and eosinophils can be observed, and when they predominate, instead of PMNs, the pattern reflects a chronic problem (Figure 6-17). ⊙

✓ Cytology results reflect nothing with respect to endometrial fibrosis, the primary reason for evaluating an endometrial biopsy.

⊙ See CD for additional cytologic images.

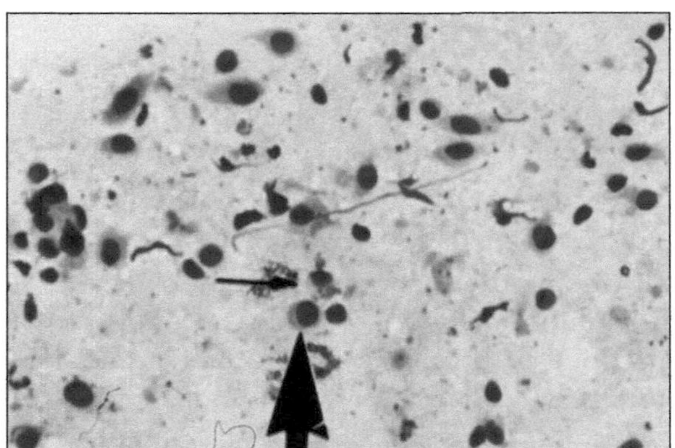

Figure 6-17 A mare's endometrial cytology pattern showing chronic-active inflammation The large arrow points to a plasmacyte and the small arrow points to an eosinophil (400x).

Endometrial Culture

✓ The discussion above on preparing the mare for obtaining the endometrial cytology applies here.

🗝 The use of a transport medium to preserve any bacteria present on the culturette is recommended. Stuart's or Amie's charcoal media are preferred.

💣 The primary inoculum should be on a solid growth medium rather than in broth which encourages overgrowth of contaminants.

⊙ The results of the bacterial culture should be reported as either no growth, or growth of a specific type or types in a qualified manner (e.g., scant, moderate, heavy) (Figure 6-18A, B, and C on CD)

🗝 Culture results must be interpreted along with and supported by other diagnostic findings or symptoms. Most pertinent and immediate would be the endometrial cytology indicating inflammation within the uterine lumen.

🗝 Accompanying inflammation within samples of an endometrial biopsy obtained at or near the same time as the culture support the significance of any bacteria isolated, but these results usually lag behind those of even a culture by 2 to 10 days.

🗝 Clinical signs of purulent or mucopurulent discharge from vulva, vagina, or cervix support the significance of culture results.

🗝 The observation of free fluid (either copious or scant) within the uterine lumen on ultrasonography tends also to support the significance of bacteria recovered on uterine culture. This finding is also directly correlated to a positive inflammatory response on endometrial cytology.

Endometrial Biopsy

🗝 The primary reason for obtaining a biopsy of the endometrium is as a prognostic tool to evaluate the mare's ability to carry her pregnancy to term.

✓ To obtain the sample the mare should be prepared as above for culture and cytology. Using similar aseptic technique, the practitioner introduces the sterile gloved hand with the sterile biopsy forceps protected in the palm of the hand through the vulva, vagina, and into and through the cervix as was performed for the culture and cytology. The biopsy forceps jaws and handle are held closed during their introduction. Once inside the uterine body they can be directed up one side or the other to obtain a sample from the left or right uterine horn. Once positioned, the practitioner removes the gloved hand from the vulva and directs it into the rectum. Palpation for the tip of the biopsy forceps is readily accomplished per rectum by following the biopsy forceps stem to the end. The handles of the forceps are rotated to 90° horizontal. As the forceps jaws are opened, the palpating hand introduces a finger into the side of the jaws and pushes endometrial tissue into their basket. The jaws are slowly closed as the finger pressure is released. The forceps is then removed from the reproductive tract, and the tissue in the forceps basket is teased out using a 20 gauge needle into 10% formalin solution, or Bouin's fixative.

💣 Samples placed in Bouin's fixative should be transferred to 70% ethanol or 10% formalin after 3-4 hours of fixation to prevent hardening of the tissue, which results in poor staining.

✓ The biopsy specimen is processed routinely and stained with hematoxylin and eosin.

🗝 Not every pathologist can interpret the histopathology of the equine endometrium adequately. Experience and training are required. It is recommended you find such a pathologist and send your samples specifically to him or her.

🗝 The most common system for endometrial histopathology classification is the modified Kenney system. This system takes into consideration inflammation and fibrosis of the endometrium and then provides an estimation of the mare's ability to conceive and maintain a pregnancy until term. The uterus is graded in the following manner:

Grade I: Basically normal with no inflammation observed and minimal, if any, fibrosis present. The prognosis for such a mare to carry a foal to term is 80-90% (Figure 6-18). ⊙

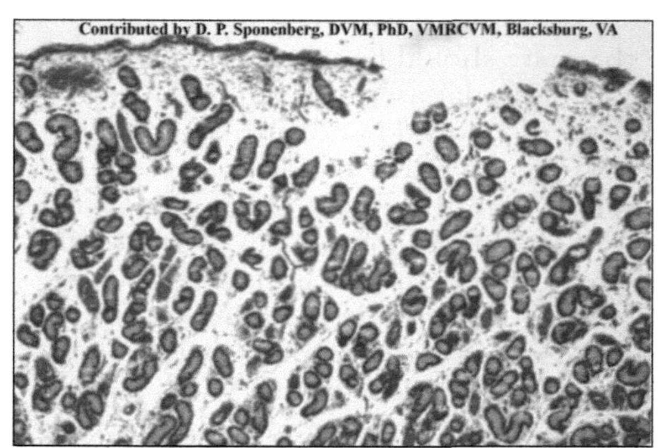

Figure 6-18
Grade 1 endometrial biopsy classification.

Grade IIA: Close to normal with some inflammatory cellular infiltrates in the stratum compactum and scattered fibrosis present throughout with some endometrial gland nesting. The prognosis for such a mare to carry her foal to term is 50-80% (Figure 6-19). ⊙

Grade IIB: Abnormal, with moderate to severe inflammatory cell infiltrates of the strata compactum and spongiosum and significant fibrosis surrounding endometrial glands causing many of them to nest together. The prognosis for such a mare to carry her foal to term is 10-50% (Figure 6-20). ⊙

Grade III: Very abnormal; active inflammation may or may not be present, but lymphocyte infiltrates will be prominent along with extensive fibrosis between and around endometrial glands causing nesting to be prominent, and some glandular lumens to be dilated; atrophy of the endometrium is also in this classification. The prognosis for such a mare to carry her foal to term is < 10% (Figure 6-21). ⊙

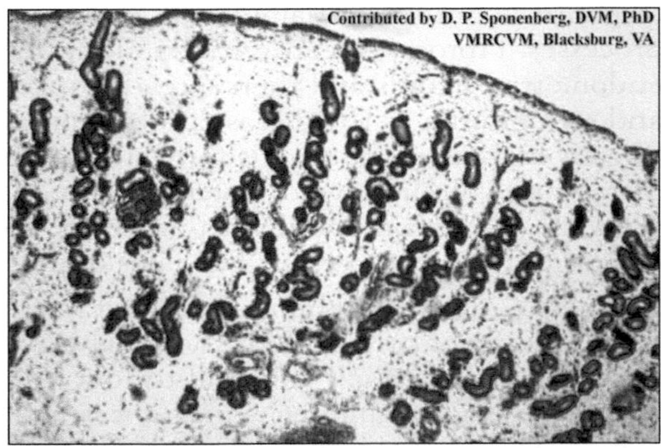

Figure 6-19
Grade IIA endometrial biopsy classification.

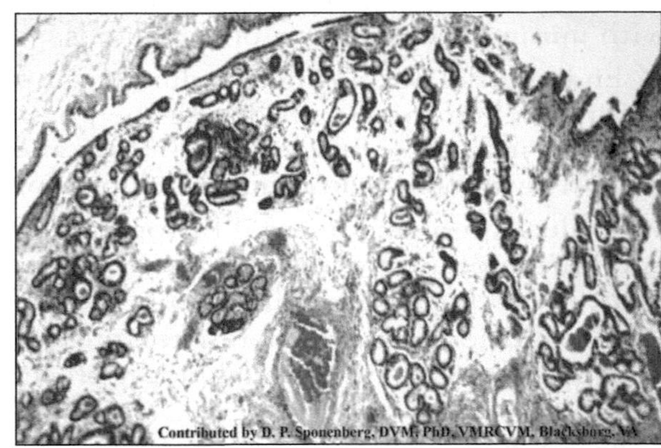

Figure 6-20
Grade IIB endometrial biopsy classification.

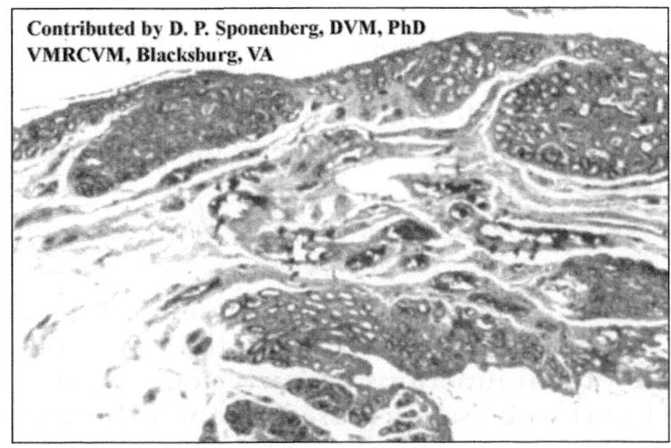

Figure 6-21
Grade III endometrial biopsy classification.

🗝 The biopsy is evaluated for the nature and severity of the inflammation. Neutrophils are seen during the acute inflammatory stages of infection; they are replaced by lymphocytes, plasma cells, and macrophages as the process becomes more chronic. Eosinophils are seen associated with fungal infections, pneumovagina, and urine pooling. Stromal cells produce collagen in response to chronic inflammation or as a result of normal aging processes. Fibrosis is seen initially along the vasculature and endometrial glands and then spreads to the stratum compactum and spongiosum as the disease process progresses. As the level of fibrosis increases, the glands form nests. Fibrosis of the basement membrane is indicative of severe disease. Dilated lymphatics (lacunae) are often noted with moderate to severe fibrosis when drainage from these vessels becomes diminished.

✓ The luminal epithelium is assessed for the presence of a continuous layer of cells and for the height of the epithelium. In estrus the cells are tall cuboidal to low columnar; these cells progress to high columnar during diestrus. The endometrial glands are straight during estrus and highly convoluted during diestrus. During winter anestrus, the epithelium is low cuboidal with minimal convolution of the glands.

✓ Endometrial atrophy occurs during winter anestrus as a normal finding. When this occurs during the physiologic breeding season, it is indicative of severe pathology and is most commonly seen in aged mares with diminished ovarian activity.

✓ Evaluation of endometrial histopathology before and after application of uterine therapy and observing response to treatment is another good application of this diagnostic procedure.

⊙ See CD for demonstration of the uterine hemorrhage that frequently follows an endometrial biopsy procedure (Video 6-4).

Hysteroscopy

✓ Transcervical endoscopic exam of the uterine lumen is an occasionally useful adjunct to diagnosis of endometrial or lymphatic cysts, foreign bodies, transluminal adhesions, and other space-occupying masses detected or suspected by rectal exam and ultrasonography.

✓ The procedure requires aseptic technique and preparation of the mare as above for cytology, culture, and biopsy.

✓ A cold disinfected (e.g., Cidex[2]) endoscope of sufficient length (1 meter) to examine the entire depth of the uterus to the uterotubal junctions on each side, and of small enough diameter (1 cm) to be safely passed through the cervical lumen is required.

[2]Johnson & Johnson Medical, Inc, Arlington, TX.

✓ Mares should be tranquilized for the procedure, restrained in examination stocks, and prepared with a full tail wrap, tail tied to the side. A perineal scrub is performed using water, cotton, and a disinfectant scrub. The operator introducing the endoscope should wear a sterile shoulder length plastic obstetrical sleeve, with a sterile non-bacteriostatic obstetrical lubricant applied to the back of the gloved hand.

✓ The tip of the endoscope is guarded by the sterile gloved hand and guided through the vulva, into the vagina, avoiding the urethral opening ventrally, and advanced cranially until the cervix is identified. The external cervical os is gently invaded and the full length of one or two fingers is inserted through the cervix, stopping at the body of the uterus. The endoscope is then carefully guided between the fingers and placed into the uterus, the lumen of which is then insufflated with air. Once the uterus is properly insufflated the examination can begin.

✓ Care must be taken not to over-inflate the uterine lumen as this may cause discomfort for the mare.

✓ The entire extent of each uterine horn should be visualized as much as possible. The blind end of each can be identified by the papilla of the uterotubal junction or ostium of the uterine tube (oviductal opening).

✓ Endometrial cysts appear as bluish to glistening gray protrusions into the uterine lumen (Figure 6-22). Endometrial cysts are typically 1-10 mm in diameter, and are dispersed multifocally

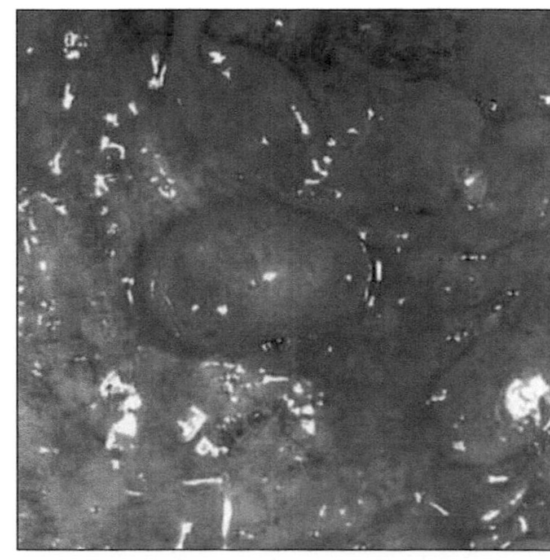

Figure 6-22 Hysteroscopic view of an endometrial cyst.

throughout one or more areas of the uterus. They result most commonly from chronic degenerative changes in the endometrium leading to periglandular fibrosis and glandular lumen restriction with dilatation of the glandular lumen resulting in its cystic distension.

✓ Lymphatic cysts are typically larger (>10 mm) and usually are isolated to one to three locations. These result from lymphatic outflow stasis. They typically have a milky or grayish-white surface appearance. Lymphatic cysts are frequently multi-loculated or compartmentalized.

Other Diagnostics

✓ A blood sample for endocrine profile or individual hormone analysis for progesterone, estradiol-17β, estrone sulfate, inhibin, or testosterone may be warranted in some circumstances.

✓ Mares suspected of having a granulosa-thecal cell tumor should have a blood sample drawn to quantify inhibin and/or testosterone.

✓ Mares examined during the breeding season but failing to exhibit signs of estrus and having no evidence of corpora lutea on ovarian ultrasonography should have a blood sample drawn to quantify progesterone and/or testosterone.

✓ Blood sampling for karyotype analysis (somatic chromosome count and sex chromosome determination) is indicated in mares exhibiting abnormally shaped or enlarged clitoris (e.g., gonadal dysgenesis).

Section 7
Breeding Management

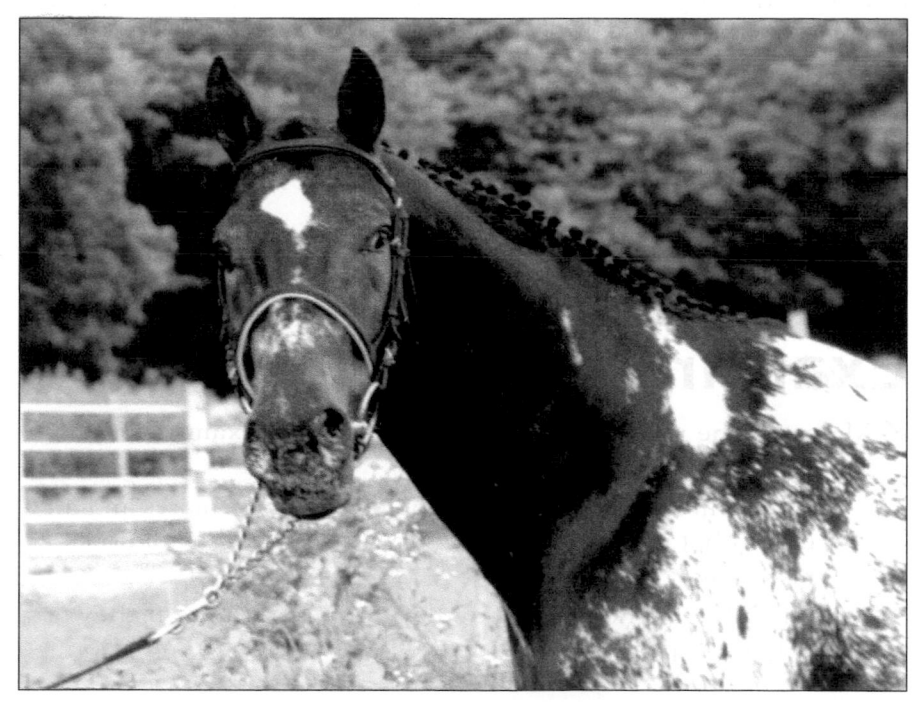

An irritable womb, with frequent straining and the ejection of a profuse secretion, may sometimes be corrected by a restricted diet and full but well-regulated work. Even fatigue will act beneficially in some such cases, hence the practice of the Arab riding his mare to exhaustion just before service. *From Law, J : Diseases of the Generative Organs. IN: Special Report on Diseases of the Horse, USDA, Bureau of Animal Industry; Washington, DC, GPO, 1916; p.174.*

Estrous Detection

✓ The success and failure of the breeding management of the mare relies heavily on determining when the mare is ready to breed according to her behavioral and physiological signs. For a discussion on teasing programs and behavioral signs of estrus, see Section 2.

✓ The mare must also be reproductively healthy prior to breeding or inseminating. For a discussion on the breeding serviceability exam, see Section 6.

✓ On large stud farms mares are teased for signs of estrus every other day.

✓ Mares showing signs of behavioral estrus should be examined for ovarian follicle development.

✓ Mares failing to exhibit signs of heat for a period of 7-10 days in a row and that are not already pregnant or awaiting their next exam for pregnancy diagnosis, should be examined to determine potential problems or to determine if she may just be shy and having 'silent' heats.

✓ The importance, efficiency, and accuracy of performing estrus detection well cannot be over-emphasized.

Examinations

✓ Mares on the roster for the days reproductive exams should include mares that:

> Are exhibiting estrus, which includes all new mares and all mares that are continuing to show estrus until ovulation is detected;
>
> Are 24 to 48 hours post-ovulation to determine if they may have post-breeding intrauterine fluid accumulation;

Are due for their initial pregnancy exam 14 to 16 days post-ovulation;

Are due for recheck pregnancy examination as determined by the practitioner's preference for interval between exams;

Have failed to exhibit signs of estrus for an interval of 7 to 10 days, and that are not already pregnant, or are awaiting initial pregnancy determination;

Have received PGF injection 2-3 days previously;

Are 2-3 days after the last day of their P4 or P+E treatment for estrous synchronization or transitional estrous management

🗝 Examinations are based on practitioner preference but rectal exam would be the minimum. Ultrasonography and vaginoscopy would be optional choices. As stated previously, this author considers it a standard of practice to combine rectal exam with ultrasonography in almost every reproductive exam.

✓ Mares with follicles ≥ 30 mm that exhibit changes in endometrial edema with a relaxed or dilated cervix are potentially close to ovulation, but may still be 2 to 5 days from this event.

✓ As follicles approach readiness to ovulate they become larger (often exceeding 45 mm in diameter), become softer or have a loss in tone or surface turgidity, and, on ultrasonography, develop increased echogenicity within their central cavity; often they point toward the ovarian fossa.

✓ Scoring of endometrial edema with ultrasound uses a subjective scale of 0 to 4.

0 = no endometrial edema evident, uterine horn cross-section is homogenous without evidence of endometrial folds; this is consistent with diestrus:

1 = very slight increase in uterine echotexture contrast; some folds may be highlighted by pockets of edema (black lines or spaces) between folds;

2 = obviously increased echogenicity of folds highlighted by edema;

3 = moderately increased echogenicity and heterogeneity; folds are well demarcated by edema having a "starfish", "wagon wheel", or "slice of orange" appearance:

4 = massive edema is present; there may be small amounts of free edema fluid within the uterine lumen as well as

between folds of endometrium; usually observed 2-3 days prior to ovulation.

✓ Changes in edema may progress rapidly from 0 to 1 or 1 to 3 over a 24 hour period of time. Most often during the final 1 or 2 days preceding ovulation there will be a reduction in the amount of edema observed.

✓ The cervix relaxes or dilates progressively as the mare enters estrus. At first it may be only 1-2 fingers in width as determined by rectal exam. In mid-estrus and usually until just after ovulation, the cervix will be 3-4 fingers in width. For a discussion on changes of the external os of the cervix as observed by vaginoscopy, see Section 6.

⦿ See CD for demonstration of ultrasound examinations of mares in estrus (Videos 7-1, 7-2, and 7-3).

Records

✓ Records help the owner, stud manager, and veterinarian to know the mare's reproductive history and patterns of change during her estrous cycles. They document findings as well as treatments. They are a must for any well-managed breeding program.

✓ The components of a good record-keeping system are as follows:

They should be complete, but too much detail a can be onerous to maintain.

They should be readily retrievable for quick review. If not their utility is lost.

They should be maintained daily as events occur. Leaving too much to memory to be recorded at a later time leads to inaccuracies or omissions.

✓ An example of the broodmare breeding record developed, modified, and used by this author can be found in Figures 7-1 and 7-2. Its advantages include ready access, a hard-copy in the barn or exam area, and sufficient details for quick review.

☝ Records may also be maintained electronically on laptop or desk top computer using one of several commercially available programs, or on a database or spreadsheet developed by the individual user. These records, as with any, should be printed to have a hard-copy for reference, and the data backed up to prevent loss of critical information.

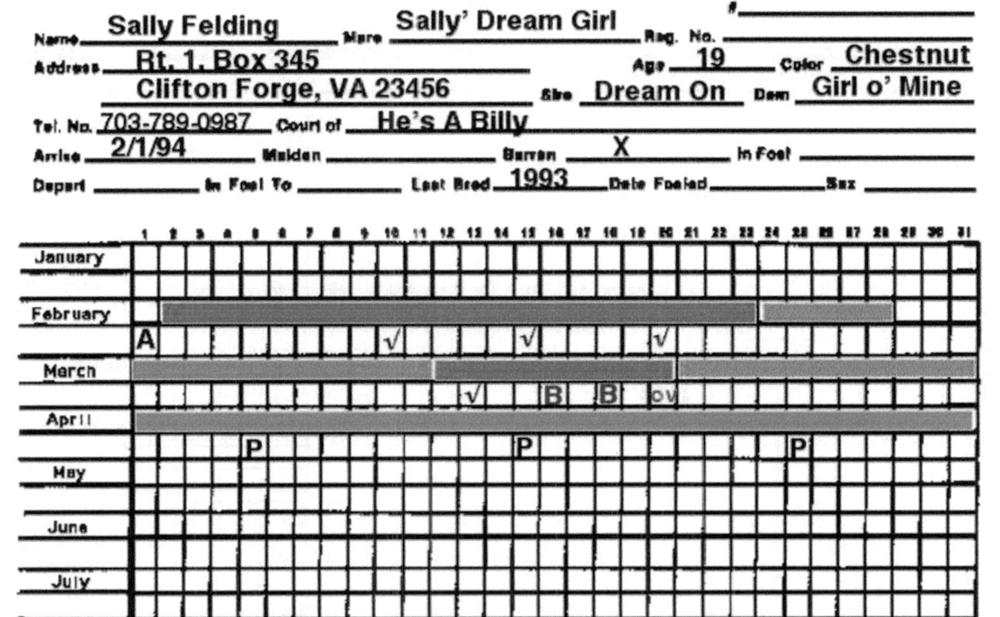

William B. Ley, D.V.M., M.S.
Diplomate ACT

MARE BREEDING REPORT

Name Sally Felding Mare Sally' Dream Girl #
Reg. No.
Address Rt. 1. Box 345 Age 19 Color Chestnut
Clifton Forge, VA 23456 Sire Dream On Dam Girl o' Mine
Tel. No. 703-789-0987 Court of He's A Billy
Arrive 2/1/94 Maiden Barren X In Foal
Depart In Foal To Last Bred 1993 Date Foaled Sex

January
February
March
April
May
June
July

Figure 7-1 Example of the breeding record I use. Mare identification and teasing history (front page). Each month is listed with consecutive days on an individual row. Red highlights stand for days of behavioral estrus. Blue highlights represent days of behavioral diestrus. Day of arrival on the farm is indicated by "A". Check marks indicate days of reproductive exam. Days of breeding or insemination are marked with a "B". Day of ovulation is marked with "ov". Positive pregnancy exams are noted with a "P".

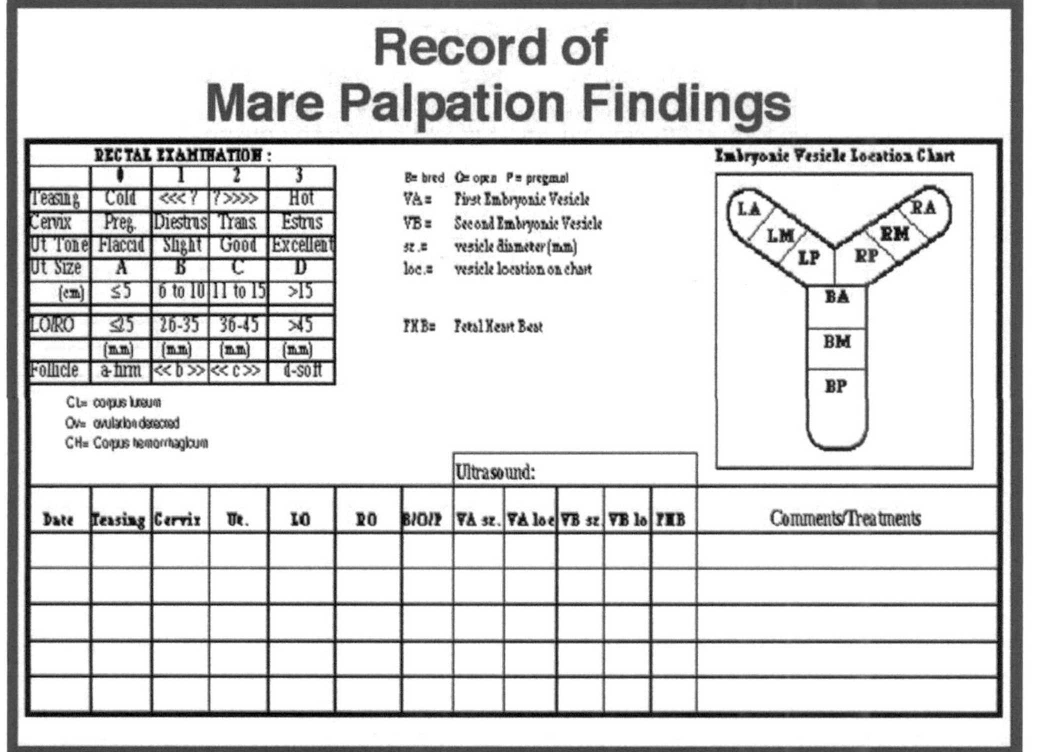

Record of Mare Palpation Findings

RECTAL EXAMINATION :

	0	1	2	3
Teasing	Cold	<<< ?	? >>>>	Hot
Cervix	Preg.	Diestrus	Trans.	Estrus
Ut Tone	Flaccid	Slight	Good	Excellent
Ut Size	A	B	C	D
(cm)	≤5	6 to 10	11 to 15	>15
LO/RO	≤25	26-35	36-45	>45
	(mm)	(mm)	(mm)	(mm)
Follicle	a-firm	<< b >>	<< c >>	d-soft

CL= corpus luteum
Ov= ovulation detected
CH= Corpus hemorrhagicum

B= bred O= open P= pregnant
VA= First Embryonic Vesicle
VB= Second Embryonic Vesicle
sz.= vesicle diameter (mm)
loc.= vesicle location on chart

FHB= Fetal Heart Beat

Embryonic Vesicle Location Chart

Ultrasound:

Date	Teasing	Cervix	Ut.	LO	RO	B/O/P	VA sz.	VA loc	VB sz	VB lo	FHB	Comments/Treatments

Figure 7-2 Example of the breeding record *I* use (reproductive exam findings on back page). The lower part of the chart is for findings on each date of exam. The table on the top left is used for shorthand values for each category on the left side. For example, palpation findings consistent with flaccid uterine tone would be marked on the chart under "Ut" as a "0". The diagram to the right represents a uterine map for designating where an embryonic vesicle or uterine cyst may be located on a particular day of exam.

Breeding by Live Cover

💣 Mares scheduled to go to the stallion should be ready to ovulate. Minimizing the number of live covers per mare per estrous cycle is good breeding practice. It also conserves stallion's resources as well as limits the amount of intrauterine challenge each mare must clear from the uterine environment before day 5-6 post-ovulation when the embryo descends from the oviduct (if she conceives).

✓ Mares susceptible to recurrent or post-breeding endometritis may benefit from a minimum contamination breeding technique (Table 7-1).

✓ Wrap the mare's tail with a bandage to incorporate all of her long tail hairs to prevent them from interfering with intromission and potentially from entangling around the stallion's erect penis and causing abrasions or even lacerations.

✓ Scrub the mare's perineum with a mild non-detergent non-disinfectant soap and rinse her very well with clean fresh water. Dry her off before proceeding to the breeding shed.

✓ Mares will preferably exhibit strong signs of receptivity to the teasing stallion to ensure a smooth cover by the breeding stallion. If not, she may need some form of mild to moderate restraint to help ensure the safety of the stallion. Such restraint may cover the spectrum from mild sedation, to application of a nose twitch, to holding or tying up one foreleg with a quick release knot, to the use of breeding hobbles. A mare in estrus and truly ready to breed should not require much convincing. But some do regardless of how ready they may be appear to be based on prior examination.

💣 Footing in the breeding shed or area should be dust free and firm enough to allow the stallion good purchase. Grassy areas serve this purpose well if not too wet or muddy. The area should be large enough to allow the mare and horse sufficient room to interact without trapping one another or their handlers in a tight spot or in a corner.

✓ The stallion should be controlled well enough to respond to his handler's requests without having to resort to too much effort to maintain control. He should approach the mare at her near shoulder or hip. Never allow him to charge directly from the rear. Courtship behavior in the wild involves an introductory period as the two approach nose-to-nose. While this is natural, it is often recommended to prevent it. Striking with a front foot by either mare or stallion is a frequent occurrence as well, which endangers the respective handlers.

Table 7-1
Minimum Contamination Breeding Technique

For Artificial Insemination Purposes	
1	The stallion is collected by sterile artificial vagina (AV) in a dust-free environment. The AV is is pre-lubricated with a sterile non-spermicidal obstetrical jelly and protected from contamination by an inverted OB sleeve until used for the collection.
2	Before the stallion is collected, he is teased and his prepuce and erect penis are washed carefully with a clean source of warm water and dried with a clean soft towel. The jump mare is prepared with a wide perineal wash and tail wrap. The phantom if used instead of jump mare is clean and dry as well. During collection the penis is directed laterally and the initial urethral secretions allowed to flush the urethra of any residual bacteria prior to application of AV and collection of the sperm-rich ejaculate.
3	After semen collection, the ejaculate is poured through a sterile filter to separate gel from sperm rich fractions into a pre-warmed (37°C) sterile container. The semen is evaluated for quality accordingly.
4	The sperm rich fraction of the ejaculate is washed by adding an equal volume of a pre-warmed semen extender with antibiotic added and centrifuged at 1500 rpm (300 G) for 3-5 minutes. The supernatant is decanted and the sperm rich pellet is gently re-suspended in warmed extender. An appropriate insemination dose is calculated and drawn up in a sterile warmed syringe which is capped, wrapped in several layers of paper towel for insulation, and then stored at 4°C for 1 hour. This gives the antibiotic in the extender time to effect a reduction of bacterial numbers in the insemination dose.
5	The mare is prepared for AI by using aseptic technique to minimize the chances of contamination of her reproductive tract and inseminated.

For Natural Service Purposes	
1	Both the mare and the stallion are prepared for breeding as described above.
2	Prior to the natural service the mare is infused with 100 ml of pre-warmed semen extender containing an appropriate antibiotic. Care is taken to minimize introduction of any air into the mare's reproductive tract (i.e., vagina and uterus) during the infusion.
3	The stallion then covers the mare naturally and ejaculates into the semen extender *in situ*.

✓ The stallion is allowed to approach the mare and tease her while obtaining a full erection. He then should be removed from her immediate environment to a neutral corner and his penis washed with mild soap and water, or just plain water. If soap is used on the stallion's penis prior to live cover it must be thoroughly rinsed to remove all residue. The penis in either case is then dried with a soft clean dry towel.

✓ The stallion is then returned to the mare in a controlled manner for the second time and allowed to take his time to mount her. Do not let him rush her from behind. An assistant or the stallion handler may sometimes need to assist the stallion in achieving intromission.

✓ Flagging of the stallion's tail is a good sign to watch for; it usually occurs during ejaculation. The stallion handler or assistant may also feel the base of the penis for urethral pulsations which also occur at this time.

💣 The stallion is allowed to take his time to dismount, but once on the ground he should be backed away quickly at a 45° angle and the mare's head should be pulled or directed towards him. This quickly decreases the likelihood that she will kick and hit him with a devastating blow.

✓ Mares may sometimes be fitted with other devices to protect the stallion from injury such as kicking boots on the rear feet.

✓ Mares may also wear protective coverings to protect them from overly aggressive stallions. A leather or heavy canvas withers cape is sometimes used to protect her from a stallion prone to biting the mare's neck when mating.

✓ Breeding horses in hand is an animated, athletic, and sometimes dangerous event. Handlers must protect themselves as well as their respective horses from injury. ⊙ See CD for demonstration of live cover breeding between the mare and stallion (Videos 7-4, 7-5, and 7-6).

Breeding by Artificial Insemination

Fresh Semen on the Farm

✓ The technique of artificial insemination is very similar to that used for obtaining an endometrial cytology or culture. See Section 6 for a complete description of the procedure.

⊙ See CD for demonstration of the AI procedure (Video 7-7).

✓ Mares susceptible to recurrent or post-breeding endometritis may benefit from a minimum contamination breeding technique (Table 7-1).

✓ Sterile disposable equipment that is non-toxic to spermatozoa is recommended for AI procedures.

✓ The optimum insemination dose for fresh extended semen is between 250-500 million progressively motile morphologically normal sperm per mare. Some farms and personnel have had successful breeding programs using insemination doses of 100 million per mare.

✓ The insemination volume ranges between 5 and 60 ml per mare. Smaller volumes have a higher risk of sperm loss, not delivering the total insemination dose needed for optimum reproductive efficiency. Volumes in excess of 60 ml in most mares typically reflux a portion of the insemination dose back through the cervix and into the vagina.

✓ Specifics of semen collection of the stallion and preparation of the semen for fresh AI on the farm will be discussed in Stallion Reproduction for the Equine Practitioner, Made Easy Series.

✓ It is preferable to use a sterile syringe with a plastic plunger for inseminations rather than one with a rubber plunger. This is especially important if the extended semen is to be stored in the syringe for more than a few minutes.

✓ The insemination is performed in the uterine body just inside the full length of the uterine cervix. A sterile insemination pipette (18–22 in.) is used. This may be introduced manually by the practitioner wearing a sterile obstetrical sleeve and a small amount of sterile non-spermicidal obstetrical lubricant. Alternatively the pipette may be passed through the relaxed or dilated cervix using a sterile vaginal speculum and light source to visualize the external os.

✓ Fresh extended semen when used for AI should be incubated at least 30 minutes (37°C) following its preparation to allow time for the antibiotic in the extender to have its full effect.

⊙ Most all extenders used for fresh AI are skim milk-based extenders. Many are commercially available as ready to use packages. The accompanying CD has a listing of suppliers for equine reproduction products and equipment, as well as some of their web sites for your ordering convenience.

✓ The chosen antibiotic included in the extender should be based on culture, sensitivity testing, and longevity testing for its potential effect for depression of the individual stallion's sperm motility.

✓ It is not critical to extend or dilute the freshly collected semen prior to AI on the farm as long as the semen will be inseminated within 10-15 minutes of collection, and provided that the total ejaculate does not have to be split among more than 3-5 mares. Extenders are an aid to splitting the volume of the ejaculate for its use in multiple mares. Dilution of the ejaculate, when it is extended, is an aid to or benefit for storage of the spermatozoa to preserve their longevity.

✓ The goal is to breed the mare 24-36 hours prior to ovulation. Fresh stallion sperm in most instances has very good intrauterine longevity. Repeat inseminations, if the mare has not ovulated, do not need to be any more frequent than once every 48 hours.

Transported Extended Cooled Semen

✓ The preparation of the mare and the specifics of the insemination are the same as for fresh insemination on the farm.

✓ Once the mare is readied, the shipping container is opened and the chilled extended semen is carefully removed. The sample is gently mixed and most of it is aspirated into an appropriately sized sterile syringe. A 1-2 ml subsample of the semen is placed in a separate sterile tube or syringe and warmed to 37°C for motility evaluation.

✓ Samples with greater than 30% progressive motility after appropriate warming can then be inseminated. If less than 30%, inquiries should be made of the stallion manager or owner as to its expected motility in an attempt to determine if there were shipping problems.

✓ Sperm motility correlates with reproductive efficiency. However, with respect to conception rate, a semen sample with 90% sperm motility is not much different than one with 50 or 60% motility. The key is in delivering an appropriate insemination dose to the mare for optimal fertility. Motility is an important component of the overall picture, but it is only a part.

✓ It is not necessary to prewarm the remainder of the insemination dose before use. Most mares are directly inseminated with the semen still chilled, which has no detrimental effect on either the sperm or the mare.

✓ See Figure 2-4 for the nondisposable shipping container most often used in North America. There are also several disposable or limited-use shipping containers commercially available. The disposable shipping containers are a cost-effective alternative to the larger more reliable nondisposable container, but their use in extremely hot shipping environments or for longer than 27-33 hours transit time should be avoided.

✓ Longevity of extended cooled transported semen once the mare is inseminated is naturally going to be shorter than with fresh semen inseminated on the farm. It has already been anywhere from 12 to 48 (or more) hours since it was collected from the stallion.

✓ The goal is to inseminate the mare once per estrus, 12 to 24 hours prior to ovulation.

✓ On occasion, more than one insemination dose per shipment is sent to the mare's owner. In this case the question arises as to what to do with the remaining dose? Is it better off in the mare? Or should it be stored for another 24 to 48 hours at 4-6°C until either used or disposed of?

✓ Most current thought is to inseminate the mare with an appropriate insemination dose upon receipt of the shipment. If too much volume is inseminated at one time the mare will reflux it retrograde. There is no proven benefit to a second insemination 24 hours later using the second dose from the original shipment.

💣 If the shipping container belongs to the stallion owner or stud farm, send it back the same day or the next business day. If not, someone may forfeit the container's deposit, and some other mare owner may not get their requested semen shipment on time, if at all!

Frozen Semen

✓ The mare should be examined for ovulation at 6-12 hour intervals once her follicular characteristics and endometrial echotexture on ultrasonography are consistent with the approach of ovulation.

✓ Preparation and insemination of the mare using frozen semen is similar to the above two procedures but with a few special considerations and some added equipment.

💣 The goal is to inseminate the mare once per estrus within 24 hours of ovulation (preferably closer to 6 hours before or 6 after ovulation).

💣 Cryopreserved and thawed stallion spermatozoa typically have a very short longevity in the mare's reproductive tract once inseminated. Some can last for 24 hours, but most have around 6 or less! For this reason, timing of insemination is much more critical using this breeding method.

✓ In most situations, the frozen semen will arrive at the mare's farm 1-3 days prior to the expected ovulation in a liquid nitrogen dry or vapor shipping container (-196°C).

💣 The semen should be accompanied by specific thawing instructions as these are not standardized like they are in the bovine frozen semen industry. Typically however, you will need at least one water bath (37°C) and a possibly a second one at 50° or 75°C plus a reliable stop watch or timer.

✓ Immediately after thawing, the semen straw is removed from the water bath, dried, loaded into the insemination pipette and the mare is inseminated. A small drop is set aside to observe post-thaw motility on a prewarmed (37°C) microscope slide.

✓ The insemination pipette may be a standard insemination pipette as used above when the semen was frozen in the larger 4-5 ml straws.

✓ When the semen was frozen in 0.25 or 0.5 ml straws and multiple straws are required per each insemination dose, the insemination instructions may specify adding the thawed sperm from each straw to a small amount of warm semen extender (37°C).

✓ Commercially available, individually wrapped, and sterile insemination guns or pipettes designed to administer either 0.25 or 0.5 ml straws may also be used.

✓ The mare should be examined 12 to 24 hours after ovulation to determine presence of post-breeding inflammation and accumulation of intrauterine fluid.

Low-dose Hysteroscopic Insemination

✓ Ensuring point of delivery as close to the site of fertilization or near the site of suspected sperm reservoir in the mare will decrease the insemination dose needed to achieve optimum conception rate.

✓ Mares inseminated near the UTJ using hysteroscopy with as few as 5 million progressively motile morphologically normal sperm have conceived at a rate similar to that for much higher sperm numbers when deposited in the uterine body by routine AI methods.

✓ The mare is prepared for routine AI as above. The disinfected endoscope (videoendoscope preferred) is inserted through the cervix and directed up the uterine horn on the same side as the expected ovulation until the papilla of the UTJ is visualized. A sterile catheter preloaded with the insemination dose is directed into the biopsy channel of the endoscope and the semen is deposited onto the UTJ, or as close as possible next to it. An air flush through the catheter follows the semen deposition to ensure that all of the insemination dose is delivered from the catheter.

✓ The advantage of this technique is particularly important to stallions with limited sperm production. It is also applicable to use of frozen semen and sex-sorted semen.

✓ One straw of a stallion's frozen semen with less than the typical insemination dose needed for standard insemination may be delivered by this technique.

✓ The advantage to the mare is that her uterus is exposed to a reduced sperm challenge. When frozen semen is used by standard AI, many mares react with an inflammatory response to the concentrated dose of spermatozoa inseminated. Use of the low-dose hysteroscopic insemination technique will circumvent this problem.

Ovulation Management

Human Chorionic Gonadotropin (hCG)

✓ 1500-3000 IU hCG can be administered intravenously or intramuscularly when the mare has a 35 to 40 mm diameter follicle.

✓ This variably assists ovulation to within the next 48-56 hours in most mares.

✓ hCG may be repeated in subsequent estrous cycles if the mare failed to conceive. There is some concern that more than two administrations of hCG in the same season may decrease its efficacy through development of antibodies to its large molecular structure. This has not been a consistent problem to many practitioners.

Deslorelin (Ovuplant™)

✓ Manufactured by Fort Dodge Animal Health, Fort Dodge, IA.

✓ This is a small (2.3 x 3.7 mm) short-acting biocompatible subcutaneous implant containing 2.1 mg deslorelin (a GnRH analog).

✓ When administered to a mare with a minimum 30 mm diameter follicle, ovulation can be expected to occur within 48 hours 80% of the time. Most hCG treated mares ovulate 48h post-treatment (range: 12-72h) while most deslorelin (Ovuplant™) treated mares ovulate 36-42h post-treatment.

✓ Packaging instructions state that it be administered subcutaneously in the neck under the mane.

✓ Treated mares have been noted to have a prolonged interovulatory interval following its use. Treated mares have suppressed LH and FSH concentrations for up to 10-14 days after ovulation.

✓ Occasionally there has been complete ovarian shutdown in a small percentage of treated mares lasting in some cases for the remainder of the breeding season.

✓ Practitioner reports indicate that administration of the implant in the submucosa of the vulva has not resulted in prolongation of the interovulatory interval.

✓ Other practitioners report that removing the implant from the subcutaneous site in the neck after the first 48 hours also eliminates any further complications in its use.

Prostagalndin-F_2 alpha (PGF)

✓ In vernal transition mares, and in mares in diestrus, PGF induces pituitary secretion of FSH and LH.

✓ Fenprostalene given 60 hours after the onset of estrus induced ovulation in 81% of treated mares vs. 31% in non-treated mares

✓ Some practitioners report observing a similar effect when using dinoprost.

Post-breeding Examination and Treatments

✓ Post-breeding endometritis is a frequent problem especially in older broodmares that have a decreased or dysfunctional uterine clearance mechanism.

✓ Every barren mare should be examined to determine the extent, if any, of intrauterine fluid accumulation 24 to 48 hours post-ovulation. This is even more critical in mares that have had intrauterine fluid accumulation noted prior to breeding.

✓ Treatment options will be discussed later in Section 10, but include uterine lavage and use of oxytocin.

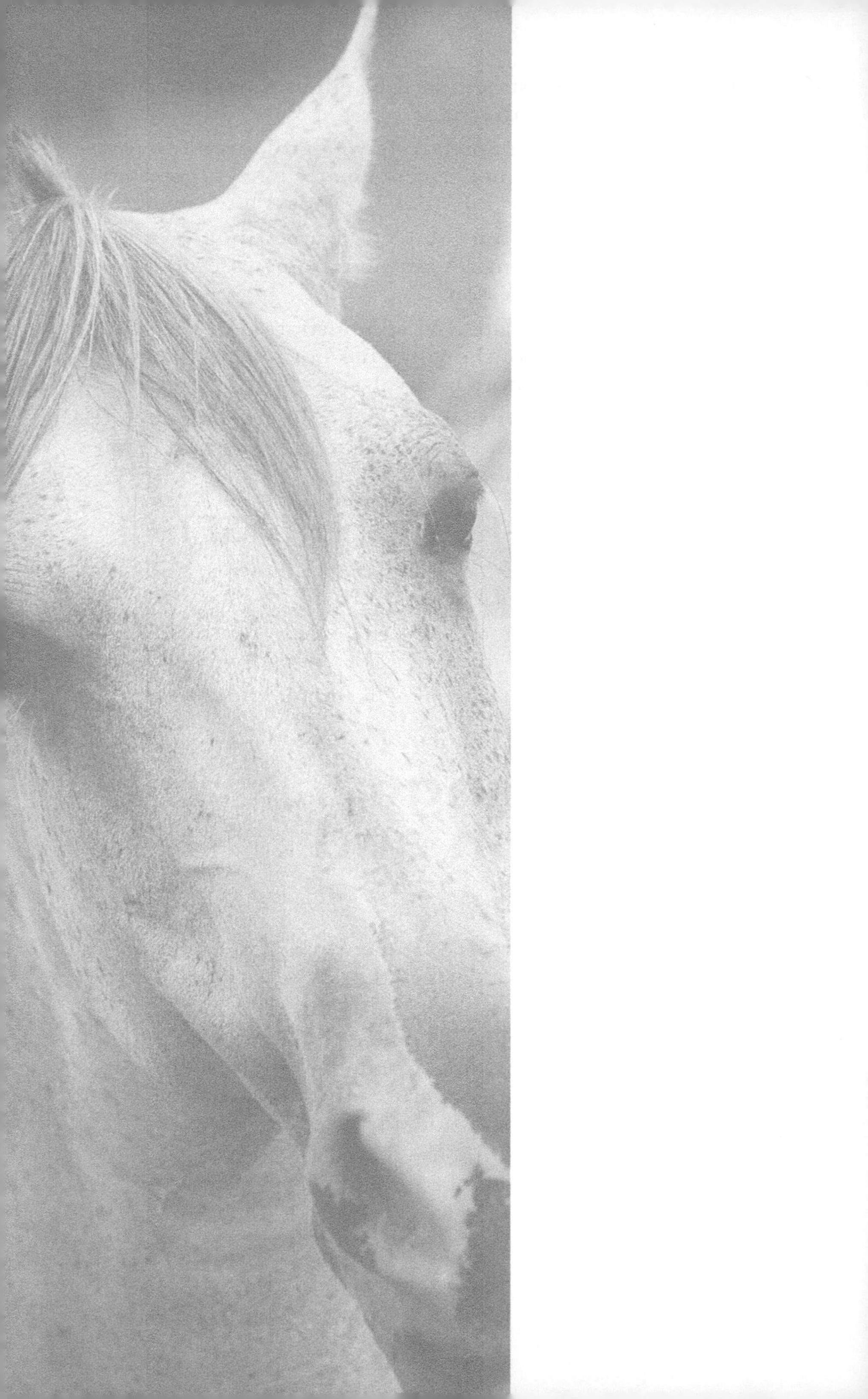

Section 8

Pregnancy Diagnosis

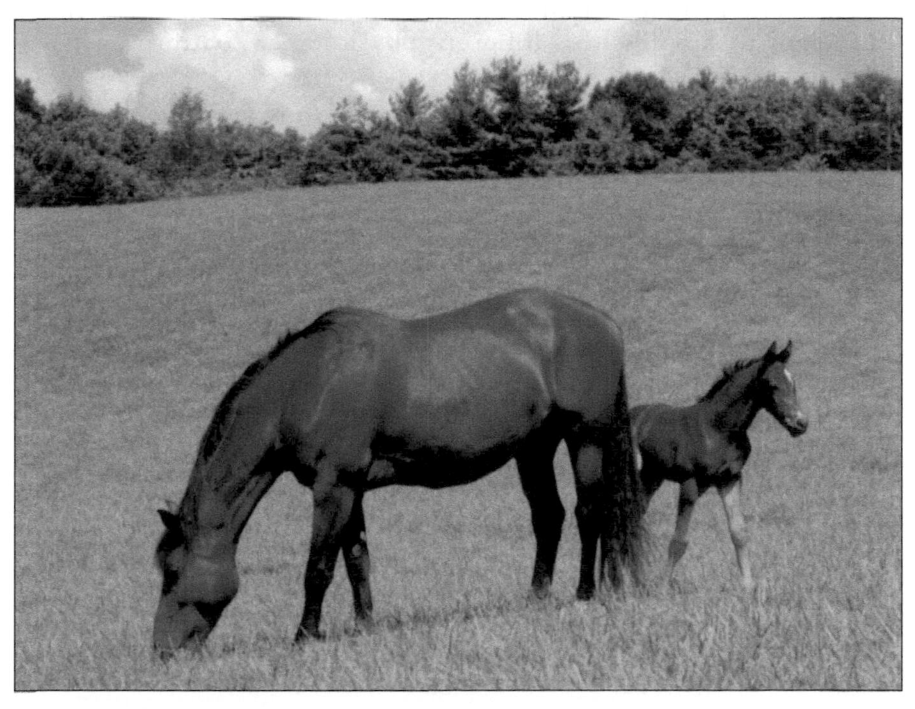

Mares failing to return to estrus following breeding or insemination are not necessarily pregnant. Failure to become pregnant may mean only that she has an active corpus luteum that is producing progesterone in sufficient quantity to keep her from showing interest in any stallion. Specific tests or examinations must be appropriately applied to determine if conception has been successful and that she remains in foal.

Behavioral Signs of Pregnancy

✓ For a review of the behavioral signs of estrus and diestrus, see Section 2.

✓ During pregnancy, the mare will most often shows signs of diestrus.

⊙ Some mares will show signs of behavioral estrus when pregnant. See CD for demonstration of teasing (Videos 2-1 and 2-2). This typically occurs between days 26 and 32 post-ovulation, corresponding to a period of follicular wave development. See Section 4 for a review of folliculogenesis. Some mares with bimodal waves of FSH secretion may have a peak in FSH around day 28 (see Figure 5-4 for a review of FSH during the estrous cycle). The primary CL and the progesterone it produces is not sufficient to suppress this inherent physiological pattern even during pregnancy.

🗝 All mares need to be teased appropriately starting between 16 and 18 days from their last ovulation/breeding. Mares showing behavioral signs of estrus at this time are most likely not pregnant. Mares not showing signs of estrus at this time may be SUSPECTED of being pregnant. But this is not a diagnosis, only a supportive sign.

🗝 Aggressive or non-receptive behavioral response of a mare to a teasing stallion is a secondary sign of pregnancy. Teasing is a screening tool to assist in breeding management. It should never be relied on as the only means of determining whether or not she is pregnant.

Vaginoscopy

💣 The characteristics of the pregnant cervix are supportive of pregnancy when viewed at the appropriate time post-ovulation/breeding. However, just as with behavioral signs it is only secondary, supportive, or suggestive of pregnancy.

✓ See Section 4 for a review of the anatomy of the cervix. See Section 5 for a review of the changes observed in the cervix when performing a vaginoscopic exam.

✓ Specifically, when observing the cervix at day 17-21 post-ovulation/breeding by vaginoscopy, the changes consistent with pregnancy include:

> The vaginal mucous membrane is pale, dry, and tacky.
>
> The external os is tightly closed.
>
> The external os is suspended centrally in the anterior vaginal fornix by dorsal and ventral frenulae.

✓ These same signs are consistent with and are not different from any non-pregnant mare under the dominant influence of progesterone secreted from a functional CL (Figure 8-1).

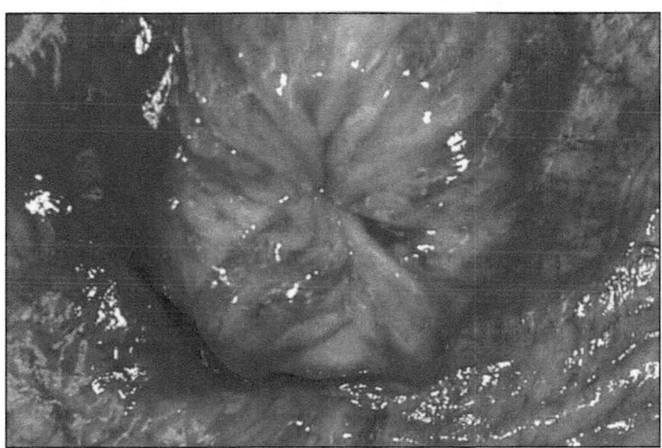

Figure 8-1 Vaginoscopic exam of the external os cervix of a mare under the dominant influence of progesterone. This can be a secondary sign consistent with pregnancy, but it should not be used as the sole diagnostic criterion.

Rectal Examination for Signs of Pregnancy

✓ To review the technique of rectal palpation of the mare's reproductive tract, see Section 6.

✓ Under most circumstances when performed by an experienced practitioner, the rectal exam is an accurate and reliable means of pregnancy diagnosis between days 17 and the last day of gestation.

✓ At or around day 17 post-ovulation (range 16-19 days), the tone and tubular character of the uterine horns increases dramatically. This is most prominent in young maiden mares and is less obvious in older multiparous mares. In some mares the tubularity almost approaches the feel of a cow's uterine horns during estrus. A sigmoid curve to one uterine horn may also be evident. The cervix is very tight and tubular and may be noticeably elongated from that noted previously during days 12-16. A palpable change in the size of one horn versus the other, indicative of the embryonic vesicle, is usually not possible except in very young maiden mares. At most there may be a gap in the degree of tone noted at the site of embryo fixation in the uterine horn.

✓ Ovarian structures may variably be palpable but are not diagnostic for pregnancy.

✓ At or around day 21 post-ovulation (range 20-25 days), the general uterine tone and tubularity will remain as described for day 17 above, but lessen to a degree. There will be a notable change in size (horn diameter) on one side indicative of the developing embryo. The change in size is noted ventrally in the horn, and will be softer in tone compared to the uterine horn areas palpable on either side. The enlargement is usually present at the base of either the right or the left horn at their junction with the uterine body. The cervical shape and tubularity will be the same as for day 17 noted above.

✓ Between days 25 and 30 of gestation, the tubularity and the tone of the uterine horns decrease and the size of the ventrally palpable bulge caused by the developing embryo increases. The palpable characteristics of the cervix are the same as for above, but it may shorten slightly in length. Ovarian changes are nondiagnostic, but there may be one or more large soft follicles palpable that may even ovulate and develop into corpora hemorrhagica (CHs) at this time.

✓ Between days 30 and 35 of gestation, little overall changes may be noted from that previously described, except that the ventrally palpable bulge of the developing embryo increases.

✓ Between days 35 and 45 of gestation, there are no further changes except the change in size of the developing embryo. Placental changes occur at this time with the development of endometrial cups that invade the endometrium, but this is not a palpable change.

✓ Palpation findings consistent with pregnancy at day 45 are sufficient to declare the mare safely in foal according to guidelines set by the American Association of Equine Practitioners (AAEP):

> *Any filly or mare shall be characterized as "pregnant" if and only if a practitioner has examined such animal for pregnancy at 42 days or more post mating during the applicable year and such examination indicated that such filly or mare was pregnant.*

✓ Between 45 and 60 days gestation, the ventral bulge of the fetus and fetal fluids inside the placenta are quite distinct and the uterine wall confining them is thin and pliant. The weight of the pregnancy carries the uterine horn into the abdomen over the pelvic brim. The non-pregnant (non-gravid) horn retains its tubularity and tone as above. As the fetal fluids expand they begin to shift across the uterine body and variably occupy part of the opposite horn. The cervix is tight and tubular but shorter in overall length.

✓ Between days 60 and 90, uterine tone diminishes even in the non-gravid side. The pregnancy can be felt more cranio-dorsal in the uterine horn and is often confused with an full urinary bladder. Careful palpation and association of structures by anatomic location will distinguish the uterus from the bladder. Tracing the fluid-filled structure caudally to a closed cervix is a key point. The fetus can sometimes be felt by ballottement within the fluid cavity of the expanded uterine horn.

✓ As the pregnancy develops beyond day 90 and its weight draws the uterus into the cranioventral abdomen, the ovaries are drawn from their normal position towards the midline and more ventral as well.

✓ Table 8-1 is a summary of the days of gestation compared with palpable changes in size and shape of the embryonic vesicle, fetus and fetal fluids.

Table 8-1
Summary of the Days of Gestation in Comparison with Palpable Changes in Size and Shape of the Embryonic Vesicle and Fetal Fluids of Pregnancy

Day of Gestation	Size of Embryonic Vesicle or Fetal Fluids	Corresponding Common Size	Crown to Rump Length
18	2.0 cm	Finger-width "gap" in tone	0.30-0.35 cm
20	2.5-3.0 cm	Bantam's egg	0.60-0.70 cm
25	3.0-3.5 cm	Golf ball	0.70-0.85 cm
30	3.0-4.0 cm	Hen's egg	0.9-1.0 cm
35	5.0 cm	Tennis ball	1.5-2.0 cm
40	6.0-7.0 cm	Lemon	2.5-4.0 cm
45-50	9.0-10.0 cm	Orange	4.0-6.0 cm
60	9.0 x 12.0 cm	Grapefruit to melon	6.0-7.5 cm
90	13.0 x 25.0 cm	Large melon to American football	10 –14 cm
110	16.0 x 30.0 cm	Rugby ball	15-25 cm
150-210	Uterus now drawn into abdomen and its outline is entirely out of reach of the examiner; fetus can be ballotted	——	30-70 cm
210 - term	Fetus easily palpable	——	

Transrectal Ultrasonography

✓ Use of transrectal ultrasonography for pregnancy diagnosis is now a standard of practice in most areas of the United States.

🗝 Its benefits include:

- Early and reliable diagnosis of pregnancy
- Detection of embryonic or fetal loss
- Early detection and management of twinning
- Gestational aging of embryo and or fetus
- Fetal gender determination
- Fetal viability determination

Pregnancy can be determined as early as 9 days post-ovulation using a 5 MHz transducer with good image resolution on the ultrasound screen.

The typical time to first attempt pregnancy diagnosis with ultrasound is day 13 to 15 post-ovulation, which is a 2 to 4 day advantage over rectal palpation alone.

The day 13 to 19 embryonic vesicle appears as a black (anechoic) spherical structure within the lumen of the uterine horn; its greatest vertical diameter (mm) closely corresponds to day of gestation from days 9 to 20. See CD for demonstration of ultrasound examinations from days 15-45 of pregnancy (Videos 8-1, 8-2, 8-3, 8-4, 8-5, 8-6, 8-7, 8-8, and 8-9)

✓ The day 18-21 day embryonic vesicle loses some of its tone and its shape as observed by ultrasound becomes triangular, or like a guitar-pick.

✓ The embryo proper can be visualized by day 20-21 and the embryonic heartbeat can be observed in real-time. Its location within the vesicle is usually between 5 and 7 o'clock.

✓ The yolk sac of the embryo recedes in size as the allantois develops. By day 24, the allantois has developed to such a point as to cause the embryo to be lifted from its ventral position. The interface between yolk sac and allantois can be seen on ultrasonography as 'wings' or faint hyperechoic lines emanating from the central embryo proper to the lateral limits of the anechoic embryonic vesicle.

✓ The embryo is seen in the center of the vesicle by day 28-30, and is near the top of the vesicle by day 35.

By day 40 the yolk sac has completely receded and the allantois is completely formed. The interface between the two join at the top of the vesicle to form the umbilicus.

✓ From day 45 to 48 the embryo suspended by the umbilicus then descends back towards the ventral aspect of the allantoic compartment.

✓ Changes in size and shape of the embryo and embryonic vesicle can be seen in Figures 8-2, 8-3, 8-4, 8-5, 8-6, 8-7, and 8-8.

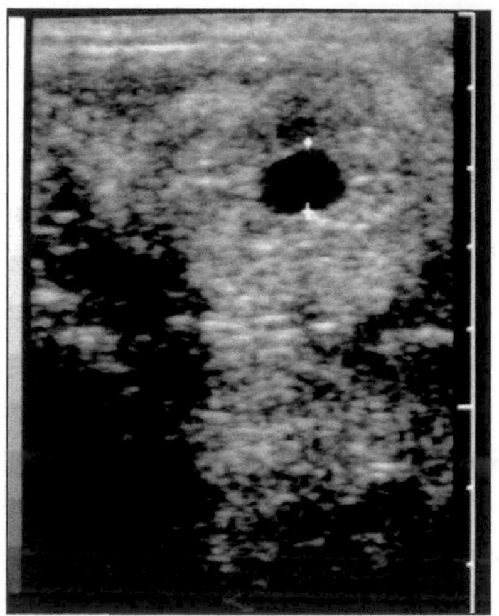

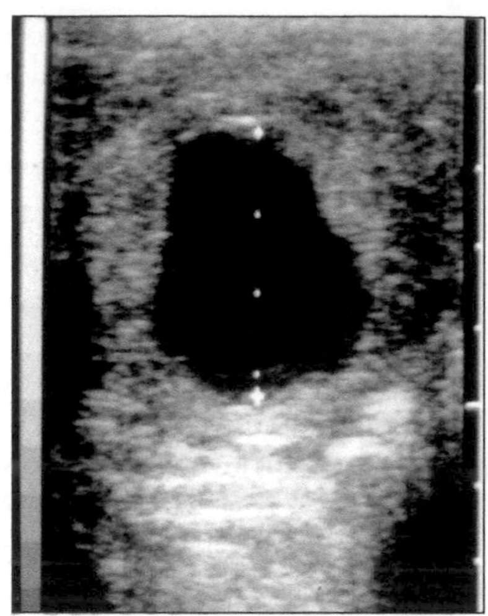

Figure 8-2 (Left) Day 14-15 embryonic vesicle as seen by transrectal ultrasonography.

Figure 8-3 (Right) Day 18-19 embryonic vesicle as seen by transrectal ultrasonography.

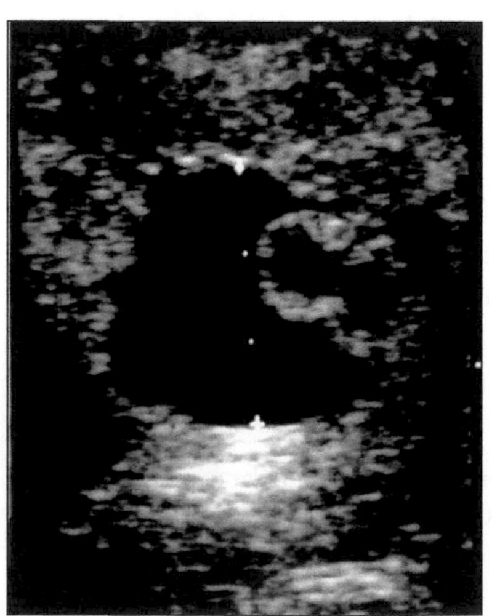

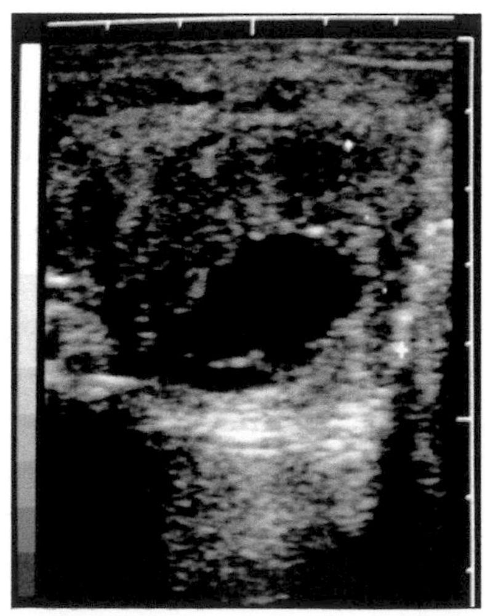

Figure 8-4 (Left) Day 21 embryo and embryonic vesicle as seen by transrectal ultrasonography.

Figure 8-5 (Right) Day 25 embryo and embryonic vesicle as seen by transrectal ultrasonography.

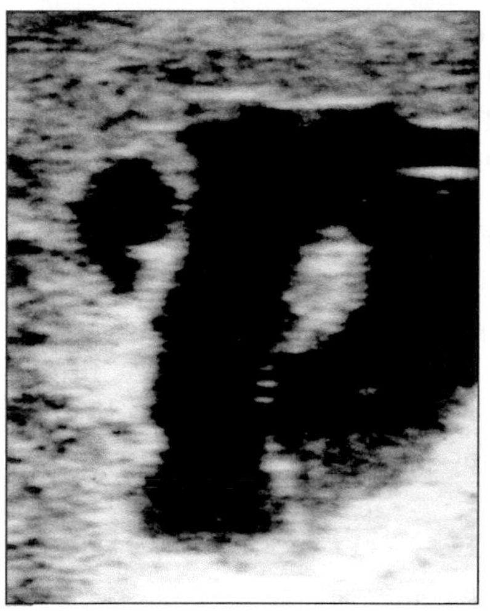

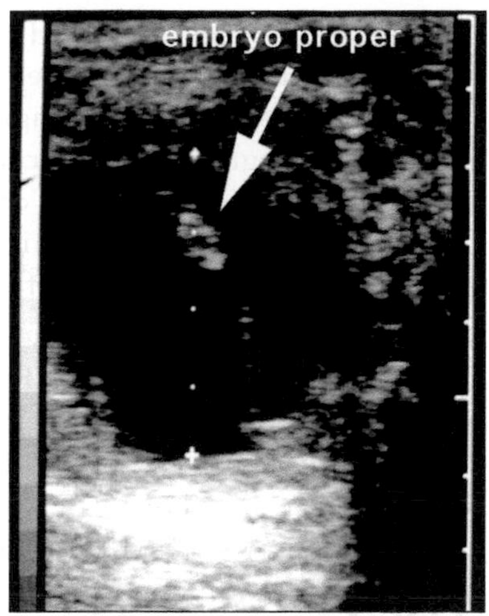

Figure 8-6 (Left) Day 30 embryo and developing placentation as seen by transrectal ultrasonography.

Figure 8-7 (Right) Day 35 embryo and developing placentation as seen by transrectal ultrasonography.

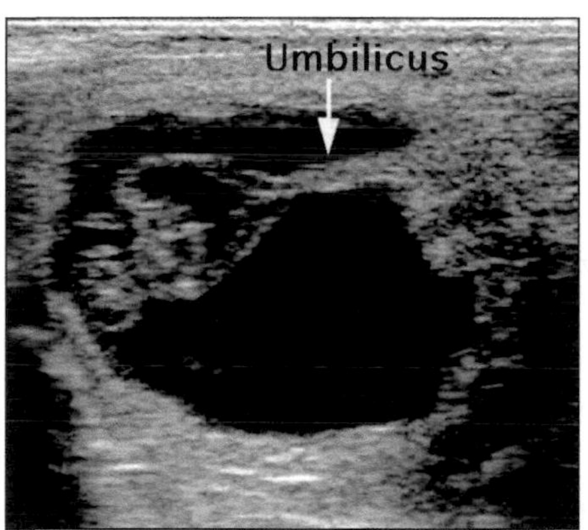

Figure 8-8
Day 45 fetus and umbilicus as seen by transrectal ultrasonography.

Hormonal Evaluations

Progesterone

✓ Serum, plasma, and milk samples may all be evaluated for progesterone levels. High values indicate simply that an active CL is producing and secreting this hormone of gestation. BUT this is not indicative of pregnancy, it is only supportive or suggestive.

✓ Blood samples obtained between days 17 and 21 post-ovulation that are high in progesterone (i.e., > 2.5 ng/ml) can be used to make a presumptive diagnosis of pregnancy. If the mare was not truly pregnant, she should not have an active CL at this time. But a late diestrous ovulation and an early embryonic loss following maternal recognition of pregnancy are confounding events that may lead to a false positive diagnosis.

⊙ Commercial kits are available for progesterone determination (e.g., ELISA or CELISA) for on the farm, or in clinic use. The gold standard for accurate measurement, however, is by radioimmunoassay (RIA). See CD for a list of suppliers and resources.

Equine Chorionic Gonadotropin (eCG, PMSG)

✓ Endometrial cup cells (i.e., trophoblastic girdle cells) invade the equine endometrium beginning around day 35-37 of gestation. Once established they quickly begin production of equine chorionic gonadotropin (eCG, PMSG). Blood levels of this hormone can be detected as early as day 42 of gestation, and usually remain elevated until around day 120.

✓ Detection of eCG by blood sampling is historical evidence that the mare was pregnant as ONLY endometrial cup cell invasion of the endometrium will cause the production of this gonadotropin.

✓ Endometrial cup cells naturally regress between day 80-120 of gestation, yet the prolongation of eCG in the systemic circulation can persist for another 20-40 days.

✓ False positive diagnoses occur when eCG levels are detected but fetal loss has occurred. Endometrial cups persist after fetal loss.

✓ False negative diagnoses occur when some mares fail to develop adequate endometrial cup invasion of the endometrium (i.e., hybrid pregnancies, and some individual mare x horse matings).

✓ In mares carrying donkey conceptuses, the chorionic girdle fails to invade the endometrium, and endometrial cups do not develop. Most of these pregnancies are aborted between days 80 and 90, but the roughly 30% that do survive and that are carried to term, do so in the absence of any demonstrable eCG.

✓ However, in donkeys carrying a hinny fetus (sire = stallion), the cups develop to a much larger size and considerably higher concentrations of eCG are achieved than in donkeys carrying a donkey fetus.

✓ There has been a sire effect demonstrated in which the amount of eCG a pregnant mare produces is influenced by the genetics of the stallion.

⊙ Commercial tests for eCG are available. Many state and commercial diagnostic laboratories offer the Equi-Check® test for PMSG (Endocrine Technologies, Inc., Newark CA 94560; 1-800-745-0843; http://www.endocrinetech.com/vet_prod.html)

Estrogens

Estrogens that are produced by the placenta of the pregnant mare and their primary metabolic by product, estrone sulfate, can be detected in plasma after day 60 of gestation.

✓ Milk samples after day 90 in pregnant, lactating mares will have demonstrable levels of estrone sulfate.

The mare is unique in production of equilin and equilenin.

The Cuboni test is historically one of the earliest hormonal assays for pregnancy used in veterinary medicine. Its basis is the detection of urinary estrogens after day 100 of gestation in the mare.

⊙ ELISA and RIA tests for estrone sulfate are commercially available and serve as a means of pregnancy diagnosis as well as fetal-placental unit health and well being. Fetal death and thus fetal-placental unit compromise result in a rapid decline of estrone sulfate concentration in plasma over a 1-3 day period of time. See CD for a list of suppliers and resources.

Tandem Hormone Assay

✓ Estrone sulfate combined with eCG can be highly sensitive and specific for pregnancy.

✓ Using this two sample technique, when eCG >1000 pg/ml and estrone sulfate > 6.0 ng/ml the sensitivity was 90% and specificity was 97% for pregnancy.

Relaxin

✓ Equine relaxin is produced by the placenta and can be detected as early as day 80, persisting until full term of gestation. It can be used as an indicator of placental health and function as well as of fetal viability and pregnancy determination.

✓ Serum relaxin concentrations are reported to range from 45-85 ng/ml in the last trimester of normal equine pregnancies. These values will decline over time in mares with problematic pregnancies.

✓ Relaxin is a protein hormone that, in various species, is thought to act synergistically with progesterone to maintain pregnancy and to promote loosening of pelvic ligaments at the time of parturition.

✓ Relaxin assays have been developed for canine serum and plasma. These have not been validated for equine plasma relaxin.

✓ Table 8-2 is a summary of equine hormonal tests that may assist in pregnancy diagnosis or fetal viability testing.

Table 8-2
Summary of Hormonal Tests That May Be Used to Assist Pregnancy Diagnosis or Fetal Viability

Days of Gestation	Test for	Sample	Comments
18 - 25	Progesterone (quantitative)	Blood or milk	Early - first indication
40 - 120	PMSG (quantitative)	Blood	Next - good indication
>60 - term	Estrone sulfate	Blood	Middle/Late - fetal placental unit viability
>80 - term	Relaxin	Blood	Middle/Late - fetal placental unit viability
>120 - term	Estrone sulfate	Fecal, saliva, milk	Middle/Late - fetal placental unit viability
>100 - term	Total Urinary Estrogens	Urine	Middle/Late - urine test

Management of Twin Conception

Twin conception occurs in 15-20% of matings in some breeds, with Thoroughbreds, Warmbloods, and draft breeds having a higher incidence. If one twin is not reduced at an early stage of gestation the usual outcome is late-term abortion of both. Twins account for 10-30% of all abortions in mares. Many complications arise with late-term abortions or delivery of twins including dystocia, retained placenta, delayed uterine involution, metritis, and death of one or both twins. Therefore, it is important that an early diagnosis of twins be made which is best done by transrectal ultrasound examination at 14-16 days of gestation.

🗝 Almost all twins are dizygotic, they arise from double ovulations. Double ovulations may be synchronous, occurring within one day of each other or asynchronous, more than one day apart.

🗝 When more than one oocyte is fertilized with a synchronous ovulation twin conceptuses of similar size are produced.

🗝 An asynchronous ovulation with double fertilization produces twin conceptuses that may vary in size up to several millimeters.

Early Intervention

✓ Between days 14-16 post-ovulation, bicornual twins (one conceptus in left uterine horn and the second in the right) can be managed by manually crushing one twin using a transrectal, ultrasound-guided procedure.

⊙ The location and size of both embryonic yolk sacs are identified in the uterus by ultrasound (Figure 8-9) ⊙, and the smaller of the two (if a size disparity is noted) is isolated and crushed between the thumb and fingers. An alternative to using the thumb and fingers is to trap the embryo to be eliminated under the flat surface of the transducer probe and against the pelvic bone applying consistent pressure until the vesicle collapses and the yolk sac ruptures (Figure 8-10). The uterus is then scanned again to verify that the remaining embryo has not been disrupted. See CD for demonstration of a twin pregnancy diagnosis at day 16 and a manual ultrasound guided twin reduction (Videos 8-10 and 8-11).

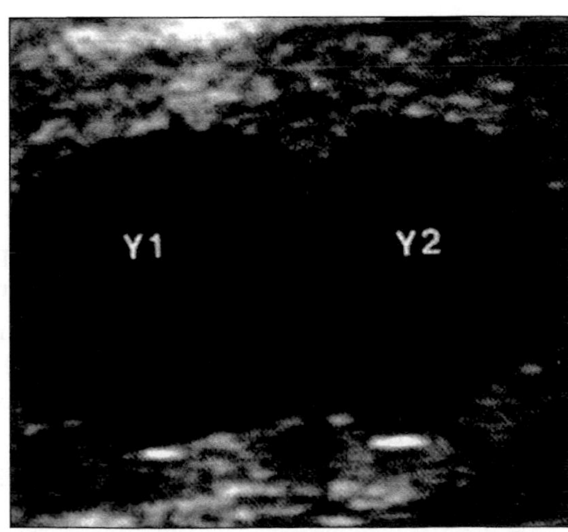

Figure 8-9 Twin equine conceptuses at day 15 are observed here in the same uterine horn (unicornual).

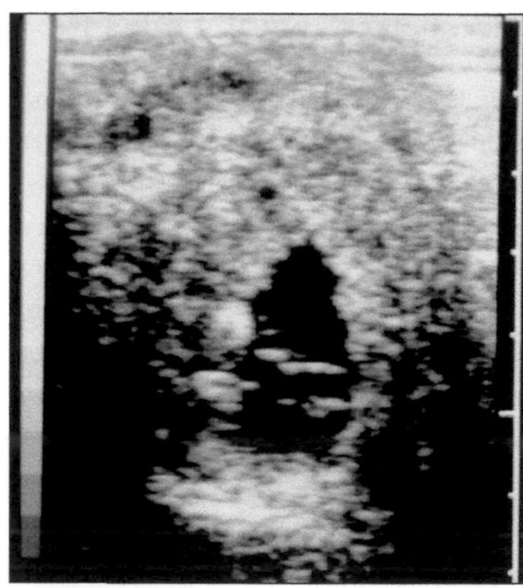

Figure 8-10 The remnants of a twin embryo are seen here after the embryonic membrane has been disrupted by manual compression.

✓ Administration of one dose of flunixin meglumine (250-500 mg, IM or PO) and 7-10 days of altrenogest (0.044 mg/kg, PO, sid) after manual reduction of one twin is suggested. The reduction may cause a release of endometrial PGF resulting in disruption of the primary CL, and potential loss of the remaining embryo.

💣 Be certain your diagnosis is correct and that you are not visualizing one conceptus and one large endometrial cyst, or two or more cysts side-by-side (see Figure 8-10, Figure 8-11 and Figure 8-12).

✓ Unilaterally fixed twins (unicornual, both in the same uterine horn, side-by-side) are more difficult to manually reduce. This intervention has a slightly higher risk of disrupting both embryos.

🔑 **The earlier that the manual intervention is performed, the better will be its success rate!**

✓ Embryos that have not yet undergone fixation (day 15-16) are more easily separated using the transducer probe and one can be manipulated to the tip of one uterine horn and crushed in that location, trapping it between pelvic bone and transducer probe.

✓ If unilaterally fixed embryos are present after day 16-17, one can still attempt to separate them with the transducer probe and isolate one embryo as above. If that fails, the option exists to wait 3-7 days and evaluate the success of natural embryo reduction.

✓ Natural embryo reduction of unicornual twins is reported to be effective in up to 85% of mares with twin pregnancy. Most natural reductions will occur before day 25, and some may not reduce until as late as days 40-45.

✓ Less than 15% of bicornual twins will reduce on a natural basis to a singleton pregnancy.

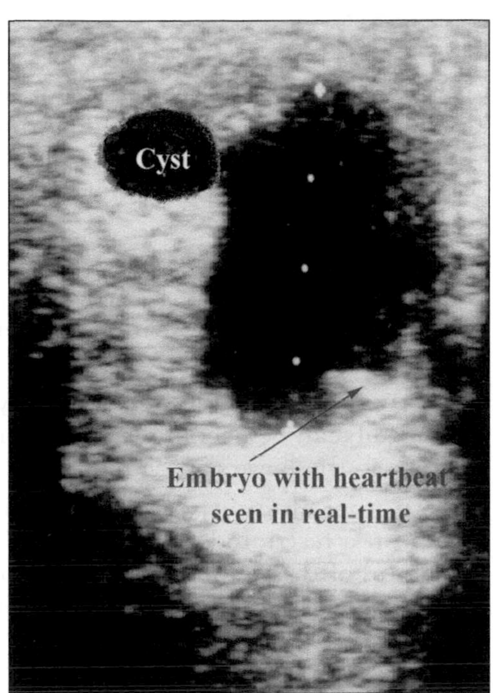

Figure 8-11 The ultrasonogram shows one embryo (day 20) and an impinging endometrial cyst.

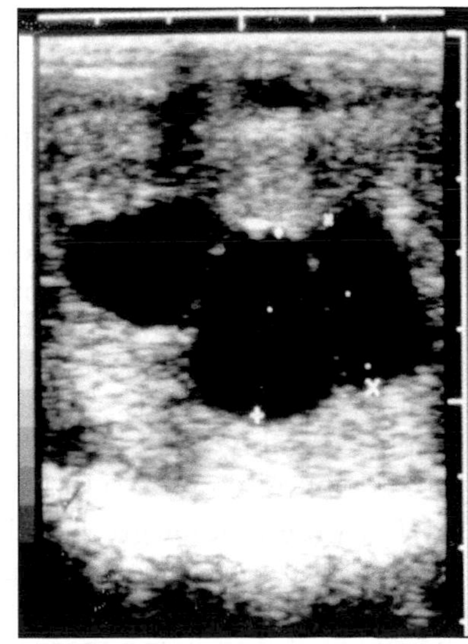

Figure 8-12 Does this ultrasonogram show triplets or two embryonic vesicles and one cyst or one embryonic vesicle and two endometrial cysts or just three cysts? How will you decide?

Late Intervention

⊙ By day 25-35 the majority of unicornual twins will be reduced by natural reduction to a single embryo (80-85% of cases), or will be undergoing visible signs of reduction. See CD for demonstration of normal singleton pregnancies at days 25 and 35 respectively (Videos 8-7 and 8-8).

✓ If both embryos have a heartbeat and are near similar in size and in opposite horns, treatment options are limited to induced abortion with PGF, continued observation and non-intervention, or allantocentesis.

✓ If there is no visible sign of embryo reduction by day 33 abortion with PGF can be accomplished before endometrial cups are functional, so the mare can be mated on the next cycle.

✓ Another alternative to active intervention is to place the mare on a restricted grass hay only diet for 14-28 days. The success rate of this technique was reported to have been 60% for mares diagnosed with twins producing single, live foals at term.

✓ Between 40 and 50 days of gestation transvaginal ultrasound-guided allantocentesis has been performed with some success. A specially designed probe for transvaginal oocyte aspiration with and end-on 5.0 or 7.5 MHz transducer probe is used for this technique. The mare is prepared as for collection of endometrial cytology or culture (see Section 6). The transducer probe is encased in a sterile obstetrical sleeve, lubricated with sterile obstetrical lubricant, and is introduced into the vagina. The operator then removes the arm from the vagina and enters the rectum to identify the uterus and embryo to be reduced. The probe head is directed to contact the embryo and its allantoic cavity with intervening walls of the vagina and uterus between. An assistant then introduces a sterile 18 gauge, 60 cm aspiration needle through the needle guide of the probe. The needle is advanced sharply to puncture all intervening structures until the allantois is entered. A 60 mL syringe attached to the needle is used to aspirate all of the allantoic fluid from the target embryo. Success rates reported have been 56% survival of the opposite embryo at 7 days after the allocentesis, and 31% survival of the opposite embryo to full term.

✓ For pregnancies greater than 60 days and up to 140 days, transabdominal ultrasound-guided fetal cardiac puncture and injection of potassium chloride (2-12 mEq) has been reported to be successful in some mares. The best window of opportunity for success using this procedure is between 115-130 days of gestation; 49% of mares with twins during this time period that underwent this procedure delivered single, live foals.

✓ Further variations on the transabdominal technique have been reported. The best success to date has been up to 62% single, live births.

✓ A final alternative for managing fetal twins is the use of exogenous progesterone supplementation along with excellent nutritional support in the hope that the mare will maintain one or both fetuses to full term. However, mares may also give birth to one full-term foal, and one mummified fetus.

Fetal Sexing

✓ Determination of fetal gender is best accomplished by transrectal ultrasonography examination between 60 and 70 days of gestation. After this time period fetal sexing is possible and diagnoses are accurate, but obtaining the appropriate view to make the diagnosis becomes more time consuming if not sometimes impossible.

✓ Fetal gender is determined by location of the genital tubercle as it migrates from between the rear limbs to near the tail in females and to near the umbilicus in males.

✓ Key points are patience, practice, experience, an optimal environment to visualize the ultrasound screen, and a high resolution ultrasound machine fitted with a 5.0 MHz transducer.

✓ See Figures 8-13 and 8-14 for representations of the male and female equine fetuses.

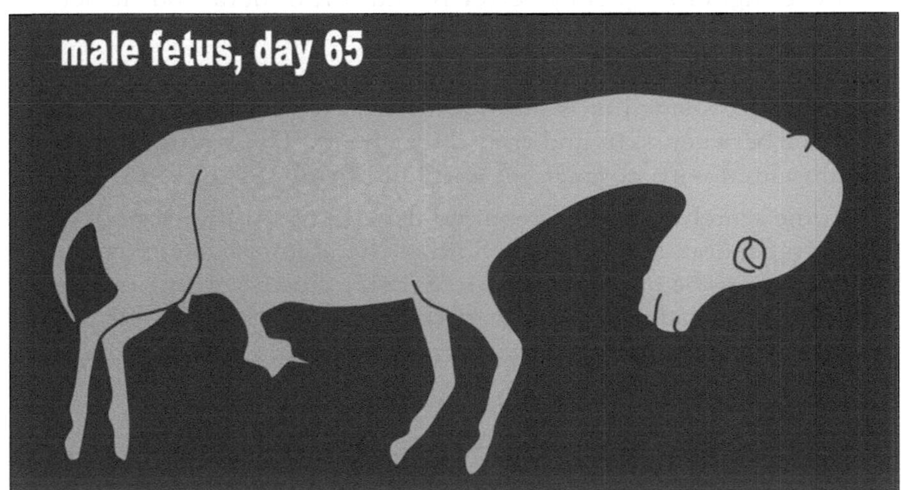

Figure 8-13 Male equine fetus at 60 days gestation

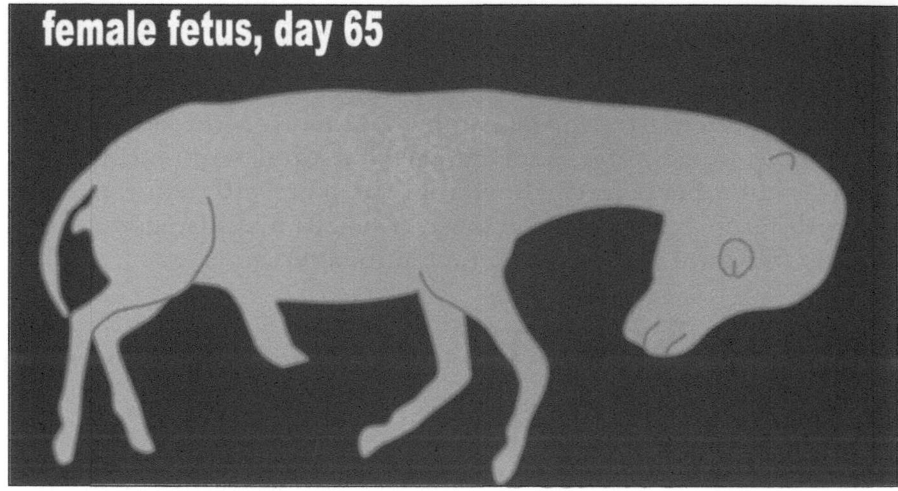

Figure 8-14 Female equine fetus at 60 days gestation.

Transabdominal Ultrasonography

✓ Pregnancy determination by transabdominal ultrasound is usually possible in mares that may be too small for rectal palpation (i.e., ponies and Miniature horses) after day 100-110.

✓ A 2.5 to 5.0 MHz transducer is recommended, the lower frequency providing greater depth of penetration but lesser detail, and the higher frequency better resolution of detail but lesser penetration.

✓ The hair of the ventral abdomen on either side of the umbilicus is either shaved or is saturated with alcohol to provide good contact between skin and transducer head. The transducer head is lubricated with contact gel and held firmly to the skin.

✓ Some searching will be required depending on the stage of gestation. In general, the anechoic fluid of the allantoic cavity is the initial sign to be observed (Figure 8-15), followed by one or more hyperechoic shadows of fetal parts (e.g., limb, head, ribs, etc.).

✓ Fetal viability is assured by observing active fetal movements or fetal heartbeat.

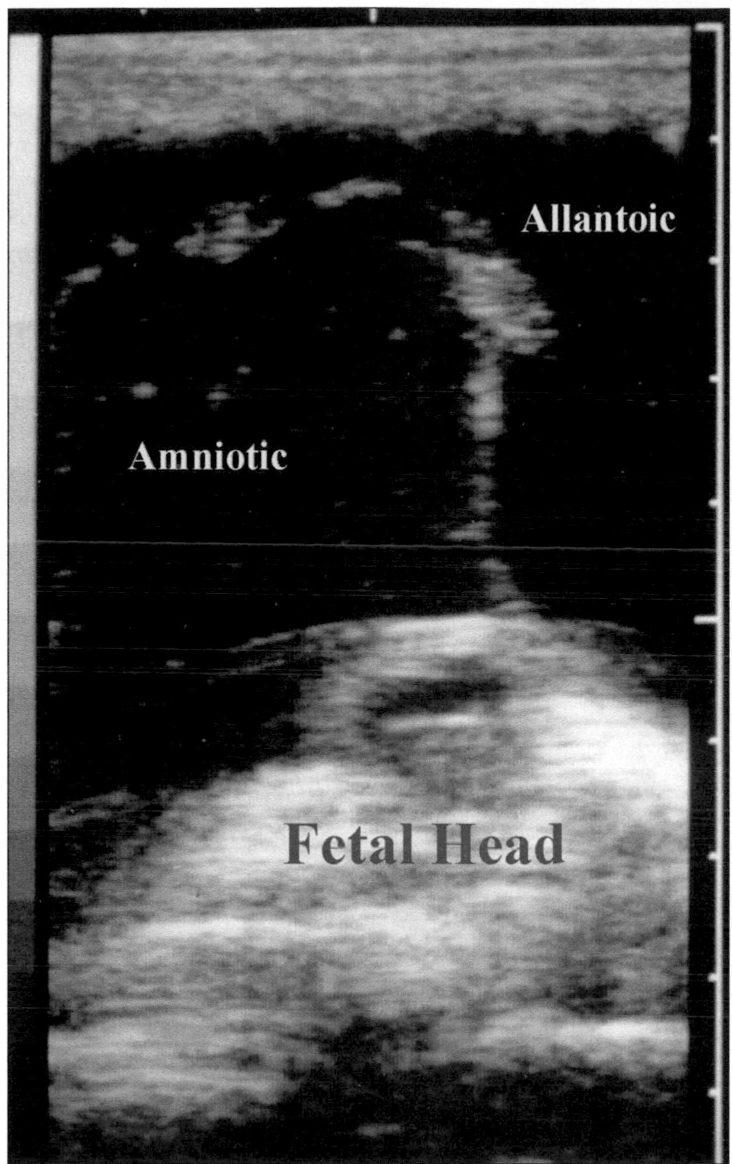

Figure 8-15 Transabdominal ultrasound of a mare that is 180 days in gestation. The allantoic fluid is anechoic. The amniotic fluid is slightly hypechoic. The fetal head and eye are observed in the bottom part of the ultrasonogram.

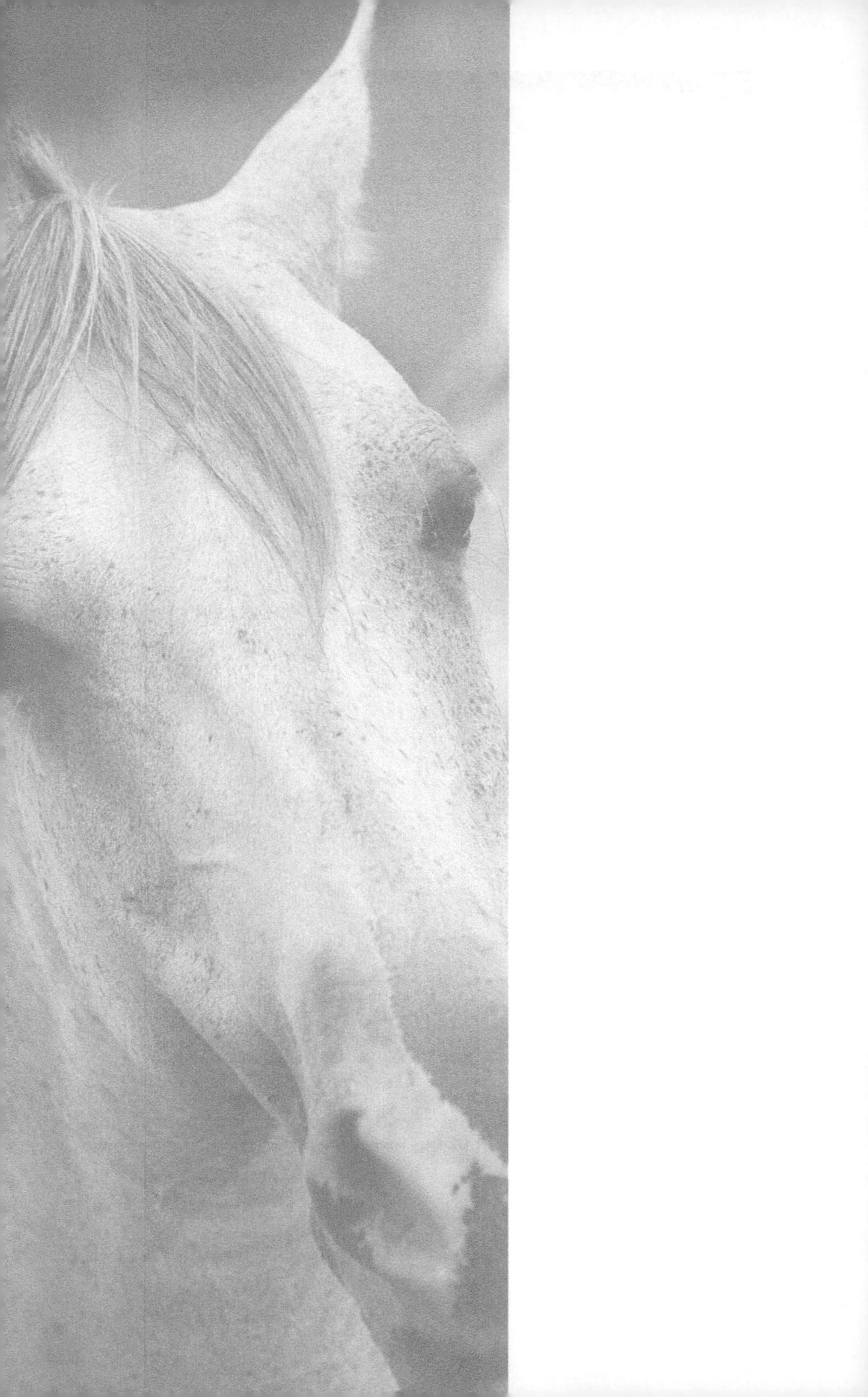

Section 9
Early Embryonic Loss

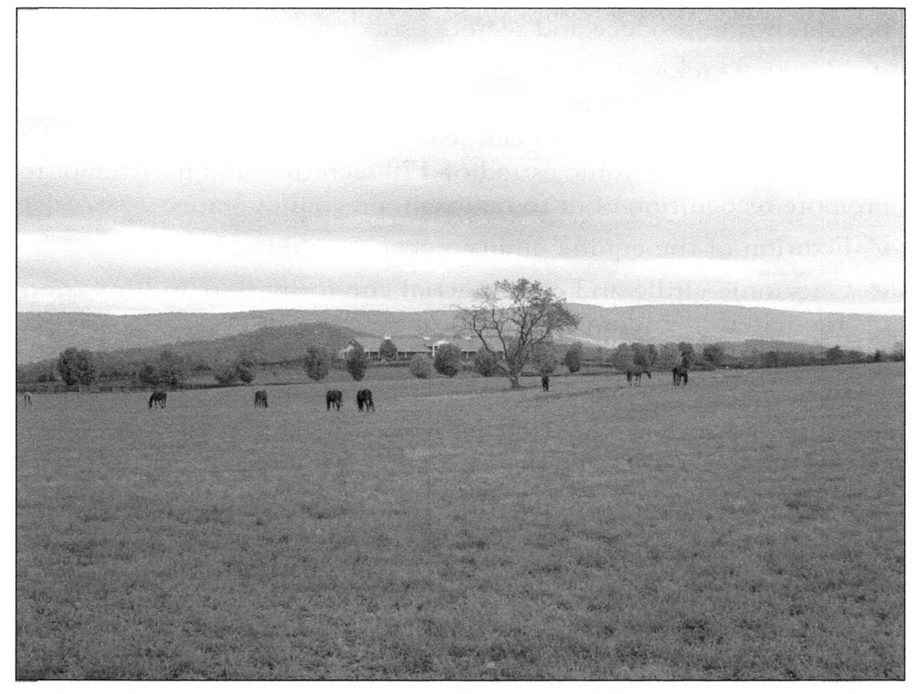

In contrast to other domestic livestock, the horse is maintained as part of the breeding population for a relatively longer period of time. In many situations, older mares may be more valuable because of their proven produce record, and it is common to find mares that are bred at greater than 20 years of age. For these reasons, age-related reproductive failure has received considerable study.

See Section 1 for a review of reproductive efficiency, rates, terms, Pregnancy, and early embryonic death (EED) losses.

Early Pregnancy Considerations

✓ The equine conceptus descends into the uterus on days 5 to 6 post-ovulation.

✓ Embryonic migration in utero occurs actively. Movement is maximal between days 11 and 14, where a complete traversal of the uterine lumen occurs every 2 hours.

✓ Embryonic contact with the majority surface area of the endometrium is necessary for maternal recognition of pregnancy and suppression of luteolysis, or promotion of luteostasis, potentially via embryonic secretion of estradiol. The equine embryo has been shown to produce and secrete estradiol-17β as early as day 12.

✓ Maternal endometrial production and secretion of PGF must be inhibited or prevented to spare the primary CL. Sufficient inflammation of the endometrium can lead to PGF release and loss of the CL overriding embryonic estradiol-17ß secretion and its attempt to promote recognition of or to maintain pregnancy status.

✓ Fixation of the equine embryo occurs on day 15 to 16.

✓ Chorionic girdle and endometrial cup formation and invasion of the maternal endometrium occur on days 35 to 37. Persistence of endometrial cups continues until day 120-130.

✓ Placental attachment begins with microcotyledonary villi interdigitation of the chorion with endometrial glands and folds by day 40 and is completed around day 70.

✓ Progesterone is required for pregnancy maintenance.

The primary CL develops by day 5-6 and persists to day 80

Secondary CLs develop around day 35-40 and persist to day 120-150.

Placental progestogen production begins around day 80 and persists to term.

The primary progestogen is pregnenolone (P5) rather than progesterone (P4).

🗝 The most important biologically active progestogen in the latter half of gestation is likely to be 5-α-pregnane-3,20-dione (5αDHP). Its key role may be in maintaining uterine quiescence.

✓ Equine chorionic gonadotropin (eCG, PMSG) is produced by endometrial cups. Secretion of eCG is detectable by day 40 and persists until day 120-150

✓ Estrogens (estradiol, estrone, estrone sulfate, equilin, equilenin):

Basal levels are present until day 90, most from ovarian sources early in gestation.

Later (after day 60) they are contributed by fetal gonads, and are metabolized by the placenta and maternal liver.

Age Related Considerations

✓ Aged mares appear to undergo a reproductive senescence characterized by lengthening of the follicular phase, irregular ovulations, and eventually follicular inactivity.

✓ The onset of these changes appears to occur over a relatively broad age range but most commonly in mares near 20 years of age or older.

✓ Prolongation of the follicular phase appears to be associated with an elevation of both FSH and LH in aged mares. The relationship of declining follicular populations, altered gonadotropin levels, and prolonged follicular development in aged mares with an increased incidence of abnormal oocytes remains to be explored as an explanation for age-related infertility in mares.

✓ Foaling rates decline with maternal age after 14 to 16 years of age. Pregnancy losses during late gestation increase in older mares due to uterine factors, but most failures of pregnancy occur early in aged mares and these account for the majority of the reduced fertility in older mares.

✓ Prior to Day 10, ultrasonographic evaluation cannot detect the early equine conceptus; however, several reports based upon embryo collection and transfer provide information regarding very early embryonic death (EED) in mares. From these studies, it appears that there is a sharp decline in the recovery rate of embryonic blastocysts from the uterus of older mares (embryo recovery attempts were performed on days 7-8 post-ovulation).

✓ Fewer embryos derived from older donor mares survive after transferring them into the uterus of reproductively healthy, younger, recipient mares. This indicates that uterine effects or environment do not play a major role in the high incidence of EED in aged mares. The impact of uterine environment may be more likely during later periods in gestation in these mares.

✓ The overall oocyte fertilization rate in young mares appears to be greater than 90%.

✓ The oocyte fertilization rate in older mares is between 80 and 90%. Thus fertilization is only slightly reduced as an effect of mare age.

✓ Estimates of EED rate between fertilization and day 10 are around 9-10% for younger mares compared with 60-70% for older mares. Most of the losses in older mares occur between fertilization and day 5-6.

✓ The effect of advancing age on reproductive efficiency in women has similarities to that of the mare:

> When intra-uterine inseminations (IUI) were performed in women between ages 40 and 42 in over 1117 cycles, only 217 pregnancies resulted, for an overall pregnancy rate of 19.4% per cycle inseminated, and a live birth rate of 12.9% per cycle inseminated. The overall live birth rate per insemination declined with advancing maternal age.
>
> The cumulative conception rate when comparing 2708 in vitro fertilization (IVF) cycles differed significantly between women 35 years of age or younger and those older than 35 years who had five or more oocytes retrieved (83% vs. 63%).
>
> There is an apparent discrepancy between the ability to maintain a regular ovulatory cycle pattern and the several years earlier cessation of female fertility.
>
> Age of oocyte donor is a significant factor influencing developmental competence of the oocyte. Age-related abnormalities of oocytes include:
>
> a. meiotic incompetence or inability to complete meiotic maturation resulting in oocytes incapable of fertilization;

b. errors in meiosis that can be compatible with fertilization but lead to genetic abnormalities that compromise embryo viability; and

c. cytoplasmic deficiencies that are expressed at several stages of development before or after fertilization

The prevailing concept of female reproductive aging in humans assumes that the decline of both quantity and quality of the oocyte/follicle pool determines an age-dependent loss of female fertility. This is largely explained by an age-related increase of meiotic non-disjunction errors leading to chromosomal aneuploidy and early pregnancy loss, so that most embryos from women 40 years old or older are chromosomally abnormal and rarely develop or implant.

✓ Few studies have addressed this issue in the horse. In one study, the in vitro maturation of oocytes from young and old mares as well as the rate of aneuploidy in oocytes from each group were evaluated. Oocytes from older mares had a delayed maturation to metaphase II compared with oocytes from young mares. Unfortunately, inadequate numbers of chromosomal spreads were available to assess the rate of aneuploidy in oocytes from these two groups of mares, and the relative incidence of aneuploidy in oocytes from aged mares remains to be defined.

🗝 Oocytes from older mares resulted in significantly fewer pregnancies than those from young mares after transfer to the uterine tubes of younger recipient mares. This study supports the evidence that an age-related decline in oocyte quality in mares is a major factor in the reduced reproductive efficiency. It appears likely that this reduction is secondary to an increased incidence of aneuploidy in oocytes from older mares; however, this remains to be established.

Uterine Tube Considerations

✓ Like the human female, the mare also experiences reproductive tract pathology of the uterine tube. This can be disappointing and costly to the mare owner, especially when it affects a proven, older, or genetically valuable broodmare.

✓ Oviductal dysfunction or pathology is a widely disputed and little understood topic in equine reproduction. A tubal blockage cannot be diagnosed through palpation, ultrasound exam, or laparoscopic examination unless a grossly obvious condition exists.

✓ Embryo transfer (ET) has been offered to owners of older mares as a potential means of producing offspring. However, a number of mares that apparently fail to conceive, may possess uterine tube abnormalities which preclude either successful fertilization (e.g., blockage of sperm transport) or embryo recovery (e.g., blockage of embryo descent into the uterus).

✓ Examination of the genital tracts from 700 mares at slaughter determined that salpingitis (inflammation of the uterine tube) does occur in the mare as determined by histopathology.

✓ Inflammation was found to occur more frequently in the ampullary region than in the isthmus, and to a greater degree, in the right side versus the left.

✓ Examination of the oviducts of 43 mares with known reproductive history found that 59% of mares in the older study group (i.e., > 7 yrs of age) had oviductal masses. Large masses were found to occupy the entire lumen of the oviduct and appeared to cause physical occlusion; such masses were greatest in number and in size from the oviducts of mares between 21-22 years of age.

✓ Pathology of the uterine tube whether it be related to physical obstruction, inflammation leading to oviductal lumen restriction or oviductal epithelial cell dysfunction may therefore be a component of EED loss in mares.

Uterine Environment Considerations

✓ The equine embryo descends from the uterine tube to the uterus between days 5 and 6 post-ovulation. The embryo at this stage is free-living, mobile, and very dependent upon endometrial glandular histotrophe secretion for its nutrient support, growth, and continued development.

✓ Endometrial inflammation and inflammatory by-products (e.g., PGF) in the uterine lumen at this stage will be detrimental to embryo survival.

✓ Contagious equine metritis caused by *Taylorella equigenitalis* commonly results in EED following initial infection in susceptible mares.

✓ Other bacteria (e.g., *Strep*, *Staph*, *E coli*, *Klebsiella*, and *Psuedomonas*) may contribute to clinical or subclinical infections and endometrial inflammation and may cause EED, but most alter placental function much later in gestation and result in abortion, stillbirth, or the birth of septic foals.

✓ Management techniques to minimize contamination of the reproductive tract at breeding or insemination are important and must not be overlooked to optimize broodmare reproductive efficiency. Some of these were discussed in Section 7 on Breeding Management, others will be discussed later in Section 10.

✓ Examination of the mare prior to and following ovulation, using ultrasonography to determine the accumulation or absence of intra-uterine fluid is a key management tool. Treatment options will be discussed in Section 10.

✓ The introduction of sperm antigens to the reproductive tract of the mare is a challenge that the mare must be able to effectively eliminate if she is to maintain conception once the embryo descends. This is even more important when considering the intra-uterine insemination of aged mares with cryopreserved semen where a high sperm antigen dose is administered in the absence of immunomodulating factors found in seminal plasma which has been removed prior to freezing.

✓ Spermatozoa initiate chemotaxis of polymorphonuclear leukocytes (PMNs) into the uterine lumen by activation of complement. Seminal plasma has been shown to down-regulate the inflammatory response and further inhibits or prevents sperm binding to uterine-derived PMNs. This effect is mediated through suppression of opsonization.

✓ Mares with a non-inflammatory uterine environment by the time the embryo descends, but having marginal or reduced endometrial glandular histomorphology (i.e., Kenney classification IIA, IIB, or III), may benefit from exogenous stimulation of endometrial glandular growth and histotrophe production using P4. Such treatments should start by day 5-6 post-ovulation to be of benefit.

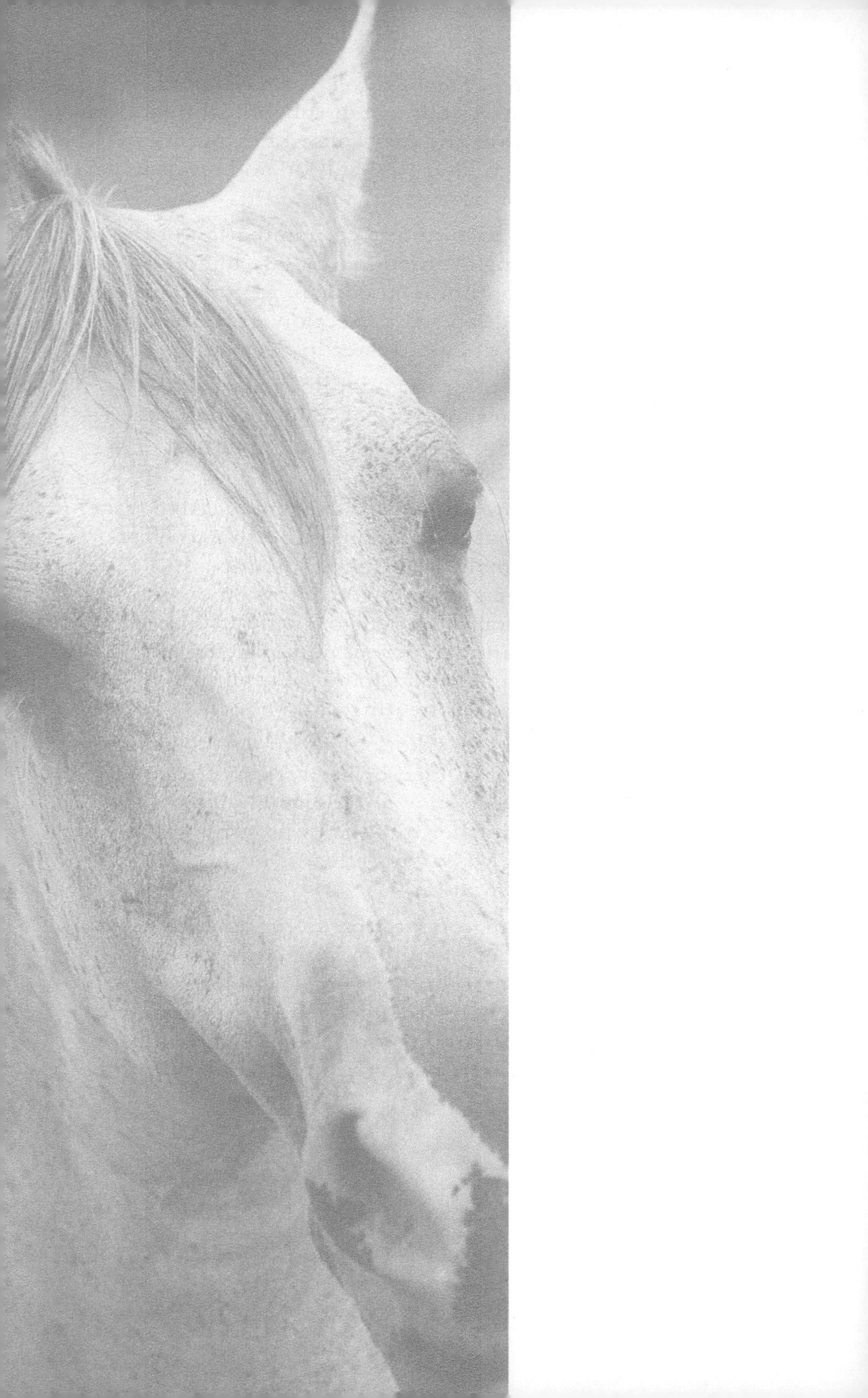

Section 10

Infectious Causes of Endometritis and Treatment Options

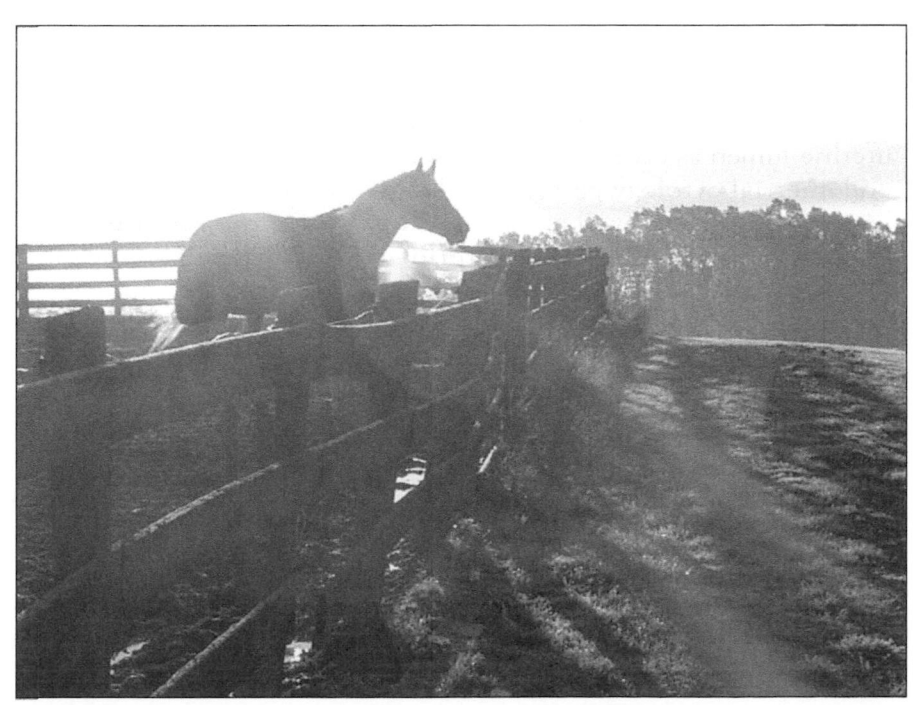

Successful treatment of the mare with acute endometritis first involves accounting for the inciting cause or causes contributing to the inflammatory condition and then controlling such factors to eliminate their recurrence. The cost, efficacy, and any potential detriments of the treatment used must also be considered.

Endometritis

Definition: An acute or chronic-active inflammation of the endometrium and its associated cellular components and structures.

✓ Typically in the mare the inflammation does not extend deeper than the endometrial layer, sparing the myometrial and serosal layers. More extensive inflammation of uterine tissues (i.e., metritis,or perimetritis) may be encountered in postpartum mares.

🗝 The following associated causes of endometritis must be considered:

- Sexually transmitted diseases
- Chronic-active or subclinical infectious endometritis
- Persistent mating-induced endometritis (delayed uterine clearance)
- Postpartum endometritis/metritis/perimetritis
- Chronic degenerative endometrosis (degenerative fibrosis)

✋ Infectious endometritis must be accompanied by signs of inflammation (e.g., purulent discharge, fluid accumulation in the uterine lumen as observed by ultrasonography, inflammatory endometrial cytology pattern, cellular infiltrates on endometrial histopathology), as well as by identification of the causative microorganism(s). A positive uterine culture by itself is not sufficient evidence.

✓ Many mares show no signs of inflammation before mating or other intrauterine challenge, but will fail to resolve the inevitable endometritis which follows such challenge(s). Breeding history is a useful indicator of such a susceptible mare. Demonstration of uterine clearance failure by use of the ultrasound to detect uterine fluid 12-24 hours post-mating/post-ovulation is most useful in practice.

✓ In many mares, the uterine fluid which accumulates prior to breeding is frequently negative on bacterial culture and contains only a few to no inflammatory cells. The importance of such fluid accumulation is that the fluid may act as a culture medium for bacteria introduced to the uterus at mating, and may in itself be detrimental to sperm survival.

✓ The amount and echogenicity of the uterine fluid observed that is considered significant is not well established. It may be that the quantity is more important than its echogenic nature. This is particularly true of fluid appearing during estrus. Generally if there is more than 1 cm of fluid within the uterine lumen observed during estrus some attempt should be made to remove it prior to breeding (e.g., oxytocin; see below with regard to uterine ecbolics). If the volume is > 2 cm, the fluid may need to be sampled for the presence of inflammatory cells and bacteria. The mare may then need to be treated by uterine lavage.

✓ Fluid observed in diestrus by ultrasonography is more serious and any detectable volume that is not pregnancy-associated, or an endometrial or lymphatic cyst, is indicative of a problem.

Endometrosis

Definition: A term used to describe the wide range of degenerative histopathologic characteristics of the endometrium of mares. This condition is degenerative (but not necessarily age-related) and lacks the typical features of active inflammation. Infiltrates of lymphocytes, plasmacytes, and macrophages are the predominating cell types observed in biopsy samples of the endometrium. There are various degrees of fibrosis in and around endometrial glandular structures, lymphatic vessel dilatation, areas of stasis, and endometrial glandular and lymphatic cysts. A development of wear and tear during the reproductively active life of the mare.

✓ Insufficient uterine blood supply, a common aging associated disorder, may play a role in the development of endometrial fibrosis and endometrosis. In older, multiparous mares, endometrial angiosis is a degenerative process affecting uterine vasculature that is a result of aging and is aggravated by multiple pregnancies. Decreased vascular elasticity can result in diminished tissue perfusion and chronic hypoxia leading to production of fibrogenic cytokines (e.g., IL-6, TNF-a, TGF-ß1), promoting fibroblast proliferation in the affected tissues.

✓ Diagnosis is based upon the mare's reproductive history and clinical examination, which includes rectal palpation, ultrasonography of the uterus, and endometrial cytology, culture, and histopathology.

Anatomic Barriers of Defense

✓ The anatomy of the perineum, vulva, vagina, and cervix are discussed in Section 4.

✓ The clinical examination of the external genitalia, vagina, and cervix are discussed in Section 6.

✓ The use of Pascoe's Caslick Index is discussed in Section 6 and illustrated in Figure 6-1. The symmetry, position, angle, and tone of the vulva and its mucous membrane apposition should all be evaluated.

✓ Additional barriers of defense against ascending microorganism invasion of the internal reproductive tract include the vestibulovaginal sphincter or seal and the cervix.

The importance of appropriate perineal conformation and preventing the introduction of external bacterial contaminants through the use of a Caslick's vulvoplasty when necessary cannot be over emphasized (Figures 10-1, 10-2, 10-3, 10-4, and 10-5). ⊙

A temporary Caslick's can be applied to the mare's vulva using a hand-held stainless steel stapling device for skin closure (Figure 10-6)⊙. Incision of the mucocutaneous junction is not performed in

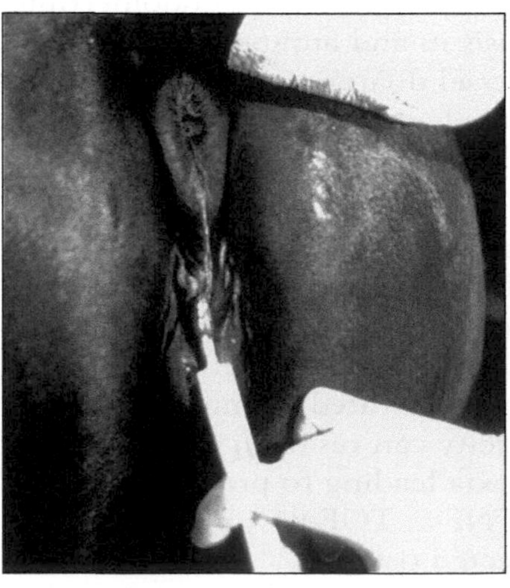

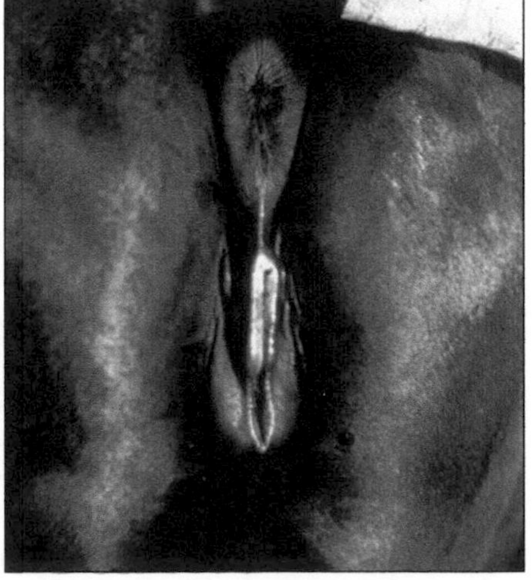

Figure 10-1 (Left) Administering local anesthesia using 2% lidocaine in a 12 ml syringe and with a 22 gauge 1.5 inch needle for the Caslick's vulvoplasty.

Figure 10-2 (Right) Showing the swelling of the muco-cutaneous junction in the vular lips following appropriate local block infiltration for the Caslick's vulvoplasty.

this technique. The staples can be removed and replaced as needed to accommodate breeding or AI and a permanent vulvoplasty performed once the mare is diagnosed safely in foal.

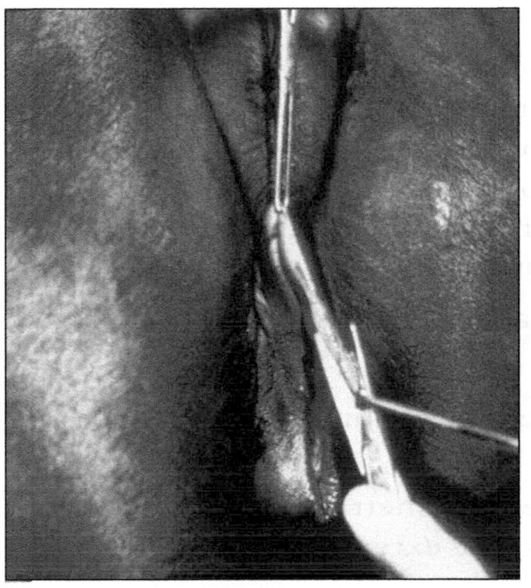

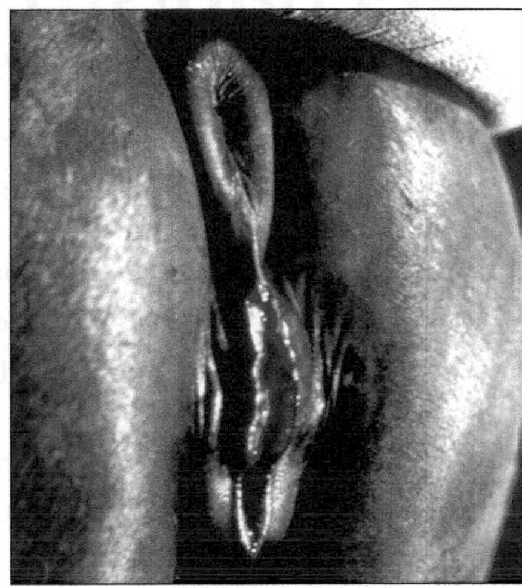

Figure 10-3 (Left) Resection of a small amount of vulvar tissue creating a surgical wound for repair by suturing during the vulvoplasty.

Figure 10-4 (Right) The surgical wound created is then sutured to bring each side of the vulva together to induce first intention healing and to reduce the effective opening of the vulva.

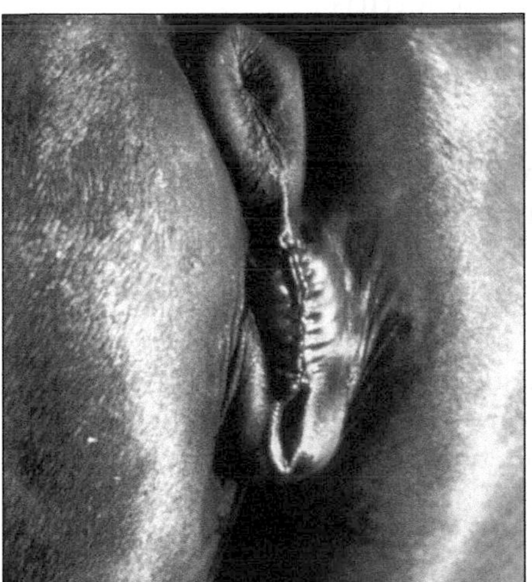

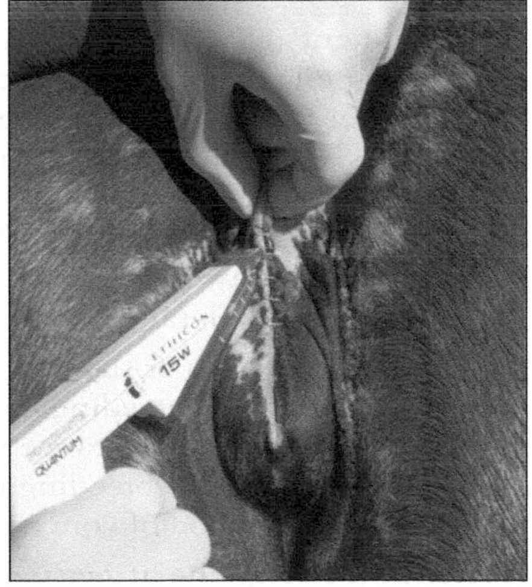

Figure 10-5 (Left) Completed Caslick's vulvoplasty in which the vulvar opening has been reduced and the suture placement sufficiently close to prevent formation of fistulas.

Figure 10-6 (Right) Demonstration of a temporary Caslick's procedure using stainless steel staples for skin closure.

Physical Clearance Mechanism

✓ Cellular (e.g., opsonins and PMN phagocytosis) and humoral (e.g., IgG, IgA and IgM) defense mechanisms against endometritis have been studied extensively. They are important in assisting the clearance of bacteria and other contaminants from the uterus, but will be ineffective by themselves if the physical clearance mechanisms are not functionally adequate.

✓ The components of the physical clearance mechanism include:

Relaxation or dilation of the cervix

Fluid secretion from the endometrium and cervix under the influence of estrogen

Rhythmic and coordinated myometrial contractions to propel uterine contents to the exterior through the relaxed cervix

Lymphatic drainage as promoted passively by myometrial activity

Impaired or dysfunctional physical clearance of uterine lumen contents appears to be the most significant problem underlying chronic or recurrent endometritis.

✓ Treatments to aid uterine clearance include nutrition, exercise, uterine lavage, and ecbolics. The latter two will be discussed later in this section. The former two are not well documented as aids to uterine clearance, but increasing general muscle tone through free exercise and the benefits of green grass (e.g., beta carotene, Vitamins A and D) will certainly not be detrimental to any mare except those with laminitis or other severe musculoskeletal disorder.

✓ Older broodmares or those considered susceptible to recurrent endometritis or post-breeding endometritis will have some compromise in their physical clearance mechanism. Adoption of a standard protocol for their breeding management will be useful in maximizing the likelihood of conception and pregnancy maintenance.

Attention to hygiene at mating/AI: Use a tail bandage, wash the mare's vulva and perineal area with clean, fresh water ideally from a spray nozzle.

At foaling: Examine all mares postpartum for the presence of trauma which might compromise the physical barriers to uterine contamination;

At all reproductive examinations: Vaginal exams should be performed as aseptically as possible; rectal exams should be followed by thoroughly washing the perineum to prevent fecal contamination of the vulva and vagina from ascending.

Correct timing of mating/AI: Minimize the number of uterine challenges the mare has to deal with. It is best if the mating or AI is performed 24-48 hours prior to ovulation. This gives one the opportunity to treat with ecbolics, uterine lavage, or intrauterine antibiotics while the mare still has an open cervix and is predominantly under the influence of estrogen.

Use ultrasound evaluation of the uterus for detection of uterine fluid in addition to conventional techniques of endometrial cytology and bacteriology, before mating/AI, and within 4-12 hours after mating/AI.

Use uterine ecbolics and lavage (see below) to promote physical clearance.

Correction of any conformational defects.

Infectious Causes of Endometritis

✓ One study from a large broodmare practice reported that in 11,922 uterine cultures, 54% resulted in no bacterial growth, 29% resulted in pure growth of a single isolate, and 17% resulted in a mixed growth of one or more isolates. All the cultures were obtained from mares prior to breeding. Can this be interpreted to mean that almost half (46%) of all mares are infected?

✓ Table 10-1 lists the most common bacterial isolates from uterine cultures.

💣 *Pseudomonas aeruginosa*, *Klebsiella pneumoniae*, and *Taylorella equigenitalis* are considered venereally transmitted diseases in the horse.

✓ Yeast and fungal organisms can also cause infectious endometritis. Reports from various laboratories indicate that fungal/yeast isolates comprise 2-3% of all positive culture results from the equine uterus. The most common of these are *Candida albicans*, other *Candida* spp., *Mucor* spp., *Saccharomyces cerevisiae*, *Hansenulla polymorpha*, *Aspergillus fumigatus*, *Rhodotorula glutinis*, *Scedosporium apiospermum*.

Yeast and fungal infections of the uterus were once thought to result primarily from overuse of intrauterine antibiotics, which is true, but this author has observed them in maiden mares never treated with any antibiotic as well in postpartum mares. They most frequently will be introduced as ascending contaminants of the reproductive tract, but occasionally can be hematogenous in origin (i.e., *Coccidioides immitus*, *Aspergillus fumigatus*)

✓ It is not uncommon for mares with mycotic endometritis to be concurrently infected with *Pseudomonas aeruginosa* or *Klebsiella pneumoniae*.

Table 10-1
The Most Common Bacterial Isolates from Equine Uterine Cultures

ORGANISM	ESTIMATED PERCENT OF TOTAL
Streptococcus zooepidemicus (+/-V)	27
Escherichia coli (+/-V)	19
Staphylococcus aureus	13
Enterobacter spp.	10
Pseudomonas aeruginosa (V)	9
Other *Staphylococcus* spp.	6
Other α- and non-hemolytic *Strep* spp.	5
Corynebacterium spp.	5
Klebsiella pneumoniae (V)	5
Taylorella equigenitalis (V)	1

(V) Venereally transmitted bacteria; (+/-V) some authors have suggested these are venerally transmitted as well.

Uterine Lavage

The definition of lavage means WASHING, especially the therapeutic washing out of an organ.

The basis for uterine lavage is to assist uterine clearance, promote uterine blood and lymphatic flow, to diminish the number of bacteria, yeast, or fungal elements that may be present, and to dilute their potentially toxic metabolic products, and to recruit or stimulate new neutrophils (PMN leukocytes) to migrate into endometrial tissues and into the uterine lumen promoting the cellular defense response.

✓ The mare is prepared for uterine lavage as she would be for endometrial cytology, culture, and biopsy as discussed in Section 6.

✓ Uterine lavage to be effective requires that a large bore flushing catheter (e.g., 80 cm, silicone, 8 mm o.d., or 33 French, with balloon cuff) or a sterile nasogastric tube (i.e., 3/8 to 5/8 in. o.d.) be used for delivery and recovery of the lavage fluid (2-10 liters) (Figure 10-7). ⊙

✓ The choice of fluid for lavage can be sterile saline (0.9% NaCl), lactated ringers solution, hypertonic saline (9% NaCl), or 0.05-1.0% (v:v) povidone-iodine solution.

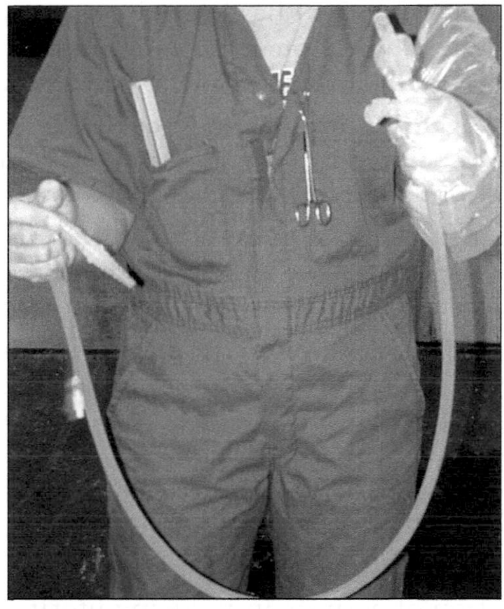

Figure 10-7
Large bore uterine catheter with balloon cuff used for uterine lavage treatment in the mare.

✓ Using aseptic technique, the practitioner guides the lavage tube through the cervix and into the uterine lumen. The lavage fluid container is connected to the lavage tubing and 1-2 liters are allowed to flow into the uterine lumen by gravity. This fluid is then siphoned back out of the uterus until as much as possible is recovered. This should be at least 90% of the volume administered, and if there were an initial amount of uterine fluid accumulated prior to the procedure it may be 100-150% or more. The procedure is repeated until the returning lavage fluid is clear or devoid of uterine debris. In some mares this may only require 1-2 liters, in others up to 10 liters may be required.

✓ The fluid temperature can be room temperature (25°C), body temperature (37°C) or warmed to 42-45°C. The higher temperatures are intended to promote uterine tone, increase uterine blood flow, and aid clearance.

Uterine Ecbolics

🗝 An ecbolic is a drug (e.g., ergot alkaloids, oxytocin, or PGF) that tends to increase uterine contractions and that were designed originally to facilitate parturition. In this discussion, I will refer to their use simply for the purpose of increasing uterine contractions.

✓ Oxytocin (20USP/mare IM or IV; range: 5 to 40 USP/mare; see Table 5-1) has been the standard choice for treating post-breeding endometritis and promoting uterine clearance.

✓ Oxytocin has been shown to have a dose-response effect with regard to uterine contractility. Lower doses 2.5 to 20 USP were associated with greater number and frequency of uterine contractions than higher doses of 30 to 40 USP.

✓ The range in onset to initial response may be from 5 to 20 minutes following its IM administration, with a mean interval from administration to initial response of 11 minutes.

✓ The duration of response is around 40 minutes for 5 units and up to 100 minutes for 40 units.

✓ Oxytocin is typically used at 5-20 USP IM or IV every 6-8 hours in the immediate post-mating or post-ovulation period for up to 24 to 72 hours. Its effect will be better if used while the cervix is still relaxed or dilated prior to ovulation.

✓ Cloprostenol (250 µg, IM; see Table 5-1) has a longer duration of activity in inducing uterine contractions (up to 90 minutes in some studies). It has been used as an alternative to oxytocin for this reason in treating mares with post-breeding endometritis. Studies have shown that it may interfere with normal CL development and progesterone production when used beyond day 2 post-ovulation.

🖐 Cloprostenol may be administered once to twice daily at 250 µg, IM, for the first 48 hours after ovulation.

Antimicrobial Therapy

🗝 The selection of an antibiotic for the treatment of infectious endometritis in the mare should be based upon appropriate uterine cytology and in vitro culture results, bacterial isolation and identification, and antimicrobial susceptibility pattern.

✓ Equally important considerations should be that the antibiotic is in an aqueous solution, does not induce a strong residual inflammatory effect upon endometrial tissues, is non-spermicidal when used near breeding or insemination, does not interfere with or inhibit uterine PMN phagocytosis, and is cost-effective.

✓ The use of antibiotic infusions to treat endometritis has had little overall impact in improving reproductive efficiency in the breeding population of mares over the past 40 years. Yet their use may significantly benefit the individual mare with an active infection.

🔑 Greater impact on improving the uterine environment and treatment of endometritis both prior to and following breeding or insemination has been obtained by the use of uterine lavage without inclusion of any antibiotic in the treatment protocol.

✓ Intrauterine antibiotic treatment intervals are usually once per day for 3 to 5 days. They may be used by themselves as a small volume infusion (e.g., 30 to 120 ml; Figure 10-8) or may follow uterine lavage therapy on each day of administration. Choices and doses for intrauterine antibiotics are presented in Table 10-2.

✓ Indwelling uterine treatment catheters have been developed to eliminate the need for constant re-entry into the reproductive tract but are only appropriate for small volume infusion therapy (i.e., 20 to 60 ml).

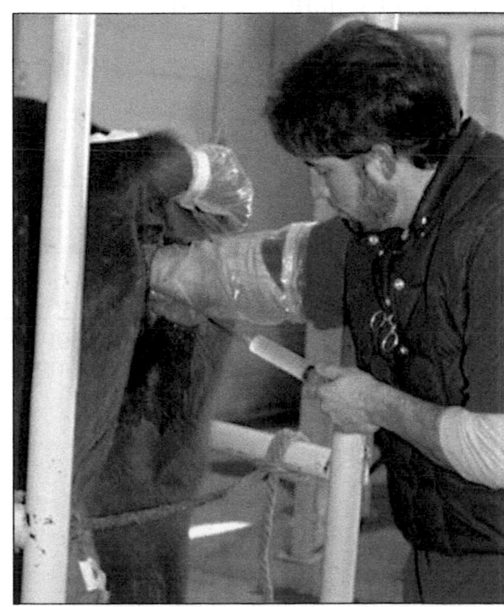

Figure 10-8 Small volume intrauterine infusion of an antibiotic is being performed.

Table 10-2
Options and Doses for Intrauterine Antibiotic Therapy in the Mare

Antibiotic	Dose	Comments
Penicillin G, Potassium or Sodium	5 Million units	Reconstitute in sterile saline or water for injection; q.s. 60-120 ml; best for *Strep. zooepdemicus*
Ampicillin, Sodium	3 g	Reconstitute in sterile saline or water for injection; q.s. 60 –120 ml
Polymixin B sulfate[a]	1 Million units	Reconstitute in sterile saline; q.s. 60-120 ml
Gentamicin sulfate[a]	2 g	Reconstitute in sterile saline; q.s. 60-120 ml; buffer with 1-2 ml 7.5-8.4% sodium bicarbonate per each gram gentamicin used
Carbenicillin	6 g	Reconstitute in sterile saline; q.s. 60-120 ml; reserve for *Pseudomonas*
Ticarcillin	6 g	Reconstitute in sterile saline; q.s. 60-120 ml; do not use for *Klebsiella*
Amikacin sulfate[a]	2 g	Reconstitute in sterile saline; q.s. 60-120 ml; may want to buffer as for gentamicin above.
Chloramphenicol sodium succinate[b]	3 g	Reconstitute in sterile saline; q.s. 60-120 ml
Ceftiofur	1 g	Reconstitute in sterile saline; q.s. 60-120 ml
Neomycin sulfate	3-4 g	Reconstitute in sterile saline; q.s. 60-120 ml

[a] Shown to inhibit PMN leukocyte phagocytosis activity in vitro.

[b] Use appropriate caution when handling and preparing due to its potential for bone marrow toxicity in humans.

✓ Systemic therapy of the mare for infectious endometritis is an option when infusions of the uterus are not possible or the practitioner determines that antimicrobial administration by this route may be preferable to intrauterine therapy. Choices for this mode of therapy are listed in Table 10-3.

Table 10-3
Antibiotics for Systemic Treatment of Mares with Endometritis

Antibiotic	Dosage	Route	Frequency
Amikacin sulfate	3.5-7.5 mg/kg	IM or SQ	bid to qid
Ampicillin sodium	25-100 mg/kg	IM or IV	tid to qid
Ampicillin trihydrate	11-22 mg/kg	IM	bid to tid
Ceftiofur	1-5 mg/kg	IM or IV	sid to bid
Gentamicin sulfate	2-4 mg/kg	IM or IV	bid to tid
Procaine penicillin G	20,000 to 50,000 IU/kg	IM	bid to tid
Trimethoprim – sulfadiazine	1.7 mg/kg - 8.8 mg/kg	IV	sid
Trimethoprim – sulfadiazine	5.0 mg/kg - 25 mg/kg	PO	sid

✓ Each invasion of the reproductive tract carries with it the risk of introducing new contaminants to the uterine environment. Minimize reproductive tract invasions or entries as much as possible in susceptible mares.

✓ Treatment of mycotic or fungal endometritis follows the same principals as for treatment of bacterial endometritis with a few extra considerations. Many laboratories offer antifungal drug sensitivity screening and where available this option should be considered to assist appropriate selection of an antimicrobial. The treatment duration should be over a longer period of time (7-14 days) compared to treatment of endometritis caused by bacteria.

✓ Available options for treatment of fungal or mycotic endometrial infections of the mare are listed in Table 10-4.

✓ Post-treatment endometrial cytology, culture, and histopathology should all be considered as part of the treatment plan.

✓ Culture and treatment of the clitoral sinus and fossa should be performed when dealing with venereal disease organisms or recalcitrant uterine infections.

Table 10-4
Options for Treatment of Mycotic Endometritis in the Mare

DRUG OR AGENT	DOSE	COMMENTS
Amphotericin B	200-250 mg	Reconstitute in sterile water; volume range from 90-120 ml; sid intrauterine infusion for 7-10 days
Amphotericin B	20 mg	Dissolve in 500 ml sterile 5% dextrose in water for intravenous administration; repeat treatment every 48h over 10 days
Clotrimazole	600 mg	Dissolve in 120 ml sterile saline; intrauterine infusion every 48h over 10-14 days
Fluconazole	150 mg	Dissolve in 120 ml sterile saline; intrauterine infusion sid for 3-5 days
Fluconazole	4 mg/kg	PO sid for 5-7 days
Griseofulvin	2.5 g	Adjunctive therapy by nasogastric tube or as a feed additive for 3 days during estrus
Miconazole	200 mg	Dissolve in 120 ml sterile saline; intrauterine infusion sid for 7-10 day period
Nystatin	0.5 – 2.5 Million units	Reconstitute in sterile water; volume range 90-250 ml for intrauterine infusion; sid for 7-10 days
Povidone iodine solution	0.05 – 1.0 % (v:v)	Volume to volume dilution of stock solution in sterile saline or water for uterine lavage; sid for 7-10 days; some mares will not tolerate povidone iodine and will develop a very irritated vaginal mucosa after 1-2 treatments
Vinegar (acetic acid)	2% (v:v)	20 ml wine vinegar in 1 liter sterile saline; for uterine lavage; sid for 7-10 days

Disinfectant Therapy

✓ The indications for use of intrauterine disinfectants or antiseptics are to reduce uterine horn diameter, increase uterine horn tone, and cause uterine irritation or inflammation.

✓ Disinfectants or antiseptics can be mild to severe endometrial irritants. The more severe their effect, the greater the likelihood of causing irreversible endometrial damage. They must therefore be used with great care and caution and with as much practitioner control as possible.

✋ Chlorhexidine solution (gluconate) should never be used as an intrauterine infusion in the mare. Chlorhexidine suspension (hydrochloride) has been used without inducing undue endometrial irritation and may be used in some cases.

✓ Mild irritants include saline (0.9% NaCl), hypertonic saline (4.5-9.0% NaCl), magnesium sulfate solution (12.8%; 12.8 g $MgSO_4$/100ml; or 1/2 cup $MgSO_4$ in a gallon of water; 42-45°C), povidone iodine solution (< 2%; v:v), hydrogen peroxide solution (25% v:v; H_2O_2), and dimethyl sulfoxide (DMSO) in concentrations less than 25% (i.e., < 25g DMSO/100ml; 7-39 mg DMSO/kg of body weight).

✓ Moderate to severe irritants include kerosene (50 ml), Lugol's iodine solution (10%; v:v), and DMSO in concentrations greater than 30% (i.e., > 30g DMSO/100ml; > 40 mg DMSO/kg of body weight).

✓ Treatment periods extend from 1 to 3 days, once per day.

✋ The goal is to induce inflammation (i.e., chemical curettage) without inducing too much endometrial damage or damage that may be irreversible (extensive fibrosis with adhesions). Inciting a small amount of irritation recruits new PMNs to the endometrium and thus the uterine lumen, increases uterine blood flow (and oxygen tension), and increases endometrial glandular secretions. The inflammatory products must be able to escape the uterus, thus an open or relaxed cervix is desirable before initiating therapy (i.e., treatments during anestrus or estrus). Uterine lavage with a non-irritant or mildly irritant fluid and use of an uterine ecbolic should be used in the follow-up period to assist uterine clearance.

🔑 The desired results of the inflammation induced are a uterus with better overall tone, smaller size, an endometrium with less (or at least not worsened) fibrosis, and elimination of chronic inflammatory cell infiltrates (e.g., small lymphocytes, plasmacytes, eosinophils, macrophages).

Alternative Therapies

Plasma

✓ Mares with chronic post-breeding endometritis may benefit from this therapy. The intra-uterine infusion of 100-250 ml fresh (heparin as anticoagulant) or frozen-thawed plasma contributes opsonins to assist PMNs in bacterial phagocytosis. However, research has shown that a relative few number of mares will actually benefit from additional opsonins to aid uterine neutrophil function.

🗝 The therapy is often preceded by uterine lavage, which may be the truly beneficial part of the treatment.

Colostrum

✓ Colostrum is rich in immunoglobulins but poor in opsonins. Its use is advocated to enhance intrauterine immunglobulins. However mares susceptible to recurrent or chronic endometritis have not been shown to have a compromised humoral defense mechanism. In fact, they have been shown to possess higher immunoglobulins in their uterine flushings when compared with uterine flushes from normal resistant mares.

Mannose

✓ Certain sugars have been shown to competitively inhibit bacterial adhesion to endometrial tissues. This has been demonstrated in vitro with equine endometrial cell cultures, as well as in vivo with intra-uterine infusion of D-mannose plus live culture of *Escherichia coli*.

✓ Controlled breeding and fertility studies using D-mannose on a large scale have not been performed but smaller scale studies have produced promising results.

✓ The treatment involves 50 g D-mannose dissolved in 1 liter sterile saline, and administering the solution as a uterine lavage therapy for 1-5 days.

✓ It is suggested that for *Pseudomonas* spp. causing endometritis the concentration be increased to 75 g D-mannose/liter.

Immunostimulants

✓ Products such as EqStim®, and Equimune®, use killed bacterial preparations that stimulate a nonspecific immune response to shorten recovery periods for infectious upper respiratory disease. They have also has been used in mares with chronic infectious endometritis and for difficult to treat cases of fungal endometritis.

✓ The active ingredient in EqStim®, is inactivated *Propionibacterium acnes*, a naturally occurring bacteria recognized as a safe yet potent stimulator of cell mediated immunity (CMI). The other ingredients in EqStim®, are USP grade ethanol and saline, providing a safe product for IV administration.

✓ The recommended dose is 1 ml per 250 lbs. of body weight. Inject the proper dose on day 1, day 3 (or 4), and day 7. After each injection, clinical signs should be monitored to evaluate the need for additional injections.

✓ Mycobacterium cell wall compounds also have immunomodulating activity. EQUIMUNE IV (Equimune,®) is an emulsion of purified mycobacterium cell walls which have been extracted by a process which reduces their toxic and allergic effects, but retains their immunostimulating activity.

✓ Equimune®, activates antigen presenting cells thereby enhancing the production of the polypeptide cytokine interleukin 1 (IL-1). The IL-1molecule is one of the body's natural adjuvants, and therefore nonspecifically amplifies the immune response to antigens.

✓ The administration of Equimune®, significantly reduced the post-breeding inflammation in both resistant mares and susceptible mares. Of special significance, Equimune®, dramatically reduced the persistent inflammation extending into diestrus of susceptible mares. The mechanism of this effect remains to be studied, but probably involves cytokines (IL1-driven, anti-inflammatory IL-10) and prostaglandin F2 alpha.

Endometrial Curettage

✓ Mechanical curettage is simple and safe to perform in the mare.

✓ When performed on 33 mares with reproductive histories of barrenness for 2 or more years, 82% showed an overall improvement in the extent and degree of chronic degenerative endometritis in their repeat biopsies following the procedure. Marked improvement occurred in 21% of the mares.

✓ Of these 33 mares, 19 produced a live foal in the breeding season subsequent to having endometrial curettage performed.

✓ This technique is safer, more humane, and has a better outcome potential than chemical curettage procedures using intrauterine irritants.

✓ The technique is best applied during diestrus. The perineum is washed as for an aseptic approach to the uterus per vaginum. The sterile curette instrument (Figure 10-9) is passed similar to the technique for performing an endometrial biopsy into the uterine body. The operator's hand is then removed from the vagina and introduced rectally. An ovary is identified and it and the ipsilateral uterine horn are stretched in a cranial direction. The curette is advanced to the tip of this horn and the operator collapses the uterine tissue closely around the base of the instrument. Multiple longitudinal strokes of the instrument are made to strip as much of the endometrium as possible from the uterine tip to the body. The same procedure is then used on the opposite uterine horn. The curettage procedure is followed by uterine lavage, and a broad spectrum intrauterine antibiotic is infused after the lavage. The uterine lavage and intrauterine antibiotics are continued for a further 4-5 days after the curettage procedure.

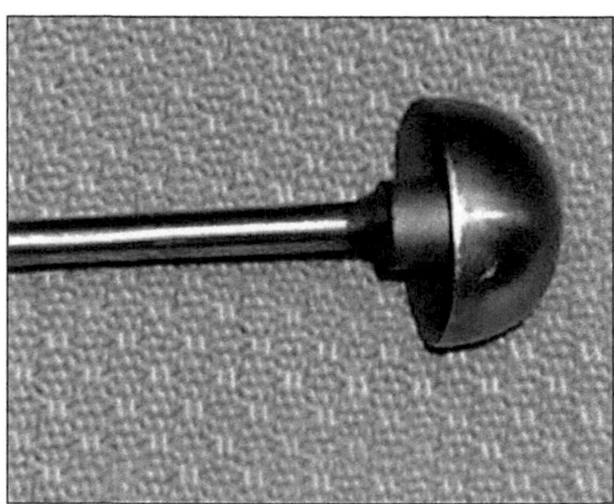

Figure 10-9 The mushroom-shaped tip of an endometrial curette instrument is depicted in this photograph. The cutting edge is on the underside of the 15 mm mushroom cap. Photograph contributed by Dr.John Dascanio VMCVM, VPI&SU, Blacksburg, VA.

Section 11

Non-Infectious Causes of Infertility

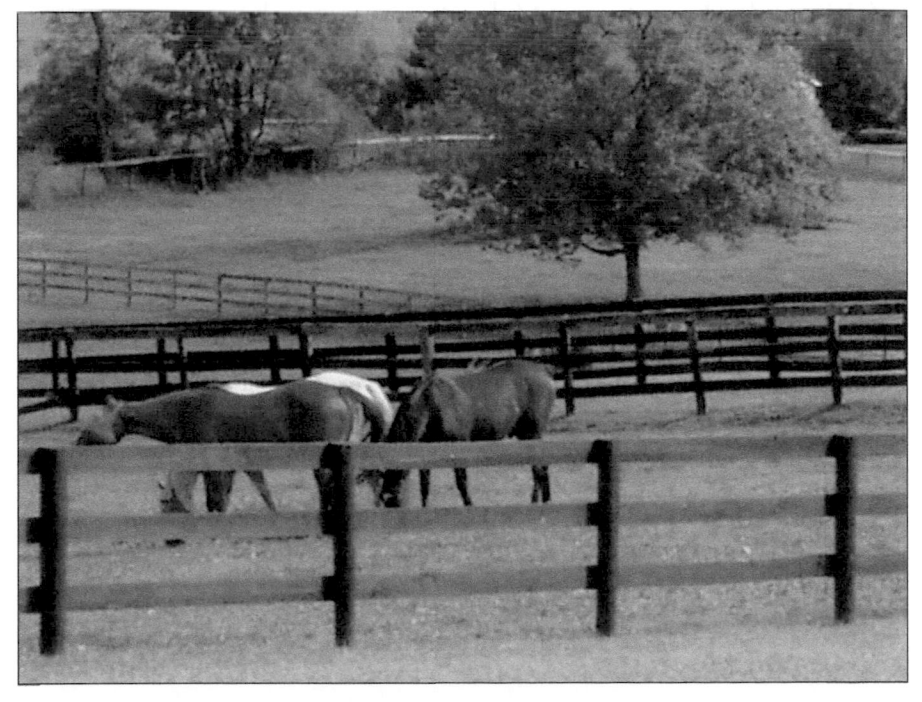

On a chromosomal basis the factors influencing infertility are complex and sometimes difficult to diagnose; infertility may be defined, biologically, as the diminished capacity for production of offspring, and statistically, as the reduction in actual numbers of offspring produced.

Cytogenetic Causes of Infertility

Definitions

✓ **Aneuploidy:** Any deviation from an exact multiple of the haploid chromosome number.

✓ The normal equine chromosome number is 64, 62 somatic chromosomes and 2 sex chromosomes; the normal stallion's karyotpe is 64XY and the normal mare's is 64XX.

✓ **Polyploidy:** Having more than two full sets of homologous chromosomes (e.g., triploid, tetraploid, etc.)

✓ **Turner's Syndrome:** Female phenotype with lack of one sex chromosome (45XO or 45X in the human, or Monosomy X)

✓ **Klinefelter's syndrome:** Male phenotype with excess of one sex chromosome (47XXY in the human, or Polysomy X)

✓ **Mosaicism:** The presence of two or more cell lines that are genotypically distinct within the same individual, derived from a single zygote.

✓ **Chimerism:** The presence of two cell lines within an individual that are of different origin as from a twin.

✓ **Trisomy:** The presence of an additional (3rd) chromosome of one type (2n + 1) in an otherwise diploid genotype (autosomal) (e.g. Down's Syndrome = trisomy 21)

✓ **Hermaphrodite:** Anomalous differentiation of the gonads with both ovarian and testicular tissues present.

✓ **Male pseudohermaphrodite:** Testicular gonadal tissues but female secondary sex characteristics; Karyotype = XX.

Etiology

✓ The complexity of gametogenesis, fertilization, and embryogenesis make meiotic errors inevitable.

✓ Meiotic or mitotic errors can cause the addition, deletion, or structural rearrangement (translocation) of one or two chromosomes in a cell resulting in aneuploidy.

✓ Fertilization errors more often involve whole sets of chromosomes, causing polyploidy.

✓ Fusions and exchanges between conceptuses of blood and germ cells produce chimeras.

✓ Mosaicism is believed to be the result of a non-disjunctional error or loss of a sex chromosome during an early cleavage division of the zygote.

Three Groups of Individuals

✓ Group I: Those rendered unable to enter, or that should be prevented from entering, the breeding population due to phenotypic heritable or physical disorder(s); offspring of heterozygous parents (carriers) for a specific defect that is expressed only in the recessive homozygous or sex-linked state.

✓ Group II: Those that possess a lethal condition within their genome that prevents their survival to reproductive age; an explanation or cause of early embryonic death or pregnancy wastage, abortions, stillbirths, and neonatal deaths.

✓ Group III: Those phenotypic individuals whose general health is essentially normal but are rendered infertile through some genotypic abnormality that specifically affects their gonads and/or internal genitalia. (e.g., intersexuality, gonadal dysgenesis, and hybrids)

Intersexuality

✓ Not a heritable condition, but probably results from chromosomal non-disjunctional errors, double fertilizations, or blastocyst fusion.

✓ Genotypic females, mosaics, or chimeras with equine karyotypes reported as 64XX, 66XXXY, 64XX/64XY, 64XX/65XY, 63X/64XX/65XXY.

✓ Equine intersexes have all been classified as male pseudohermaphrodites. They possess hypoplastic male gonads or ovotestes with an enlarged, penis-like clitoris and male libido; karyotype is 64XX (Figures 11-1, 11-2, and 11-3). ⊙

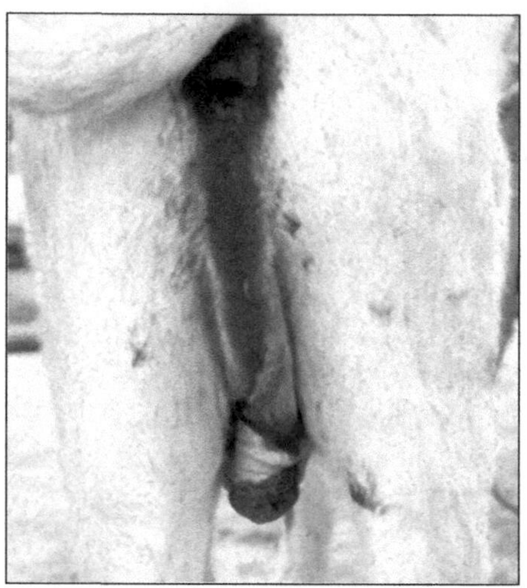

Figure 11-1 Posterior view of a male pseudohermaphrodite (MPsH) with rudimentary penis directed ventrally between the rear legs and located caudal to the scrotum.

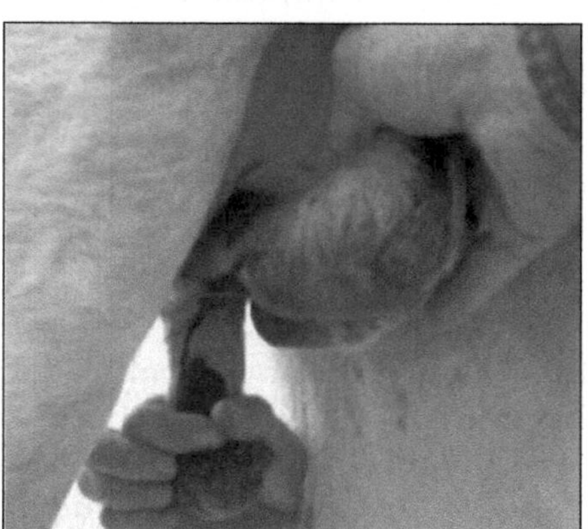

Figure 11-2 The same MPsH in Figure 11-1 showing the relationship between penis and scrotum. Tail is to the left of the photo and head is to the right.

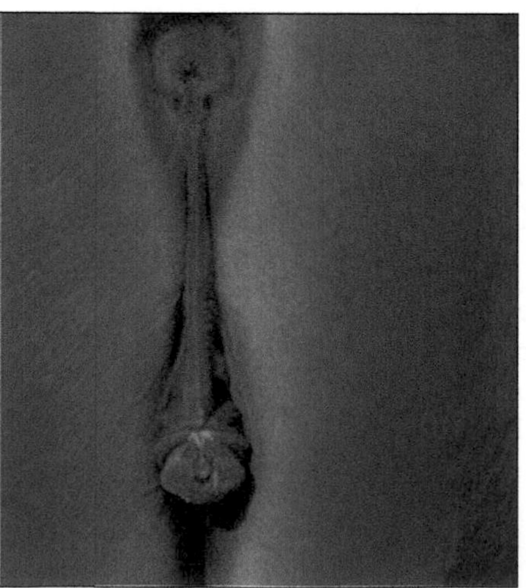

Figure 11-3 A filly presented with the primary complaint of an enlarged clitoris. This horse was another MPsH.

Polymorphonuclear leukocyte screening for 8 to 12% expression of X-chromatin condensation, or a "drumstick" on the nuclei of PMN-leukocytes is rapid and reliable indication of XX-female genotype (i.e., Barr bodies).

Chromosomal analysis (karyotyping) can be performed on fresh blood collected into a vacuated tube containing either acid citrate dextrose or heparin as an anticoagulant. The sample should be sent by overnight courier to a laboratory capable of animal karyotyping. Several are listed in Table 11-1, along with their web sites.

✓ Surgical gonadectomy and phallectomy or clitorectomy (as the case may be) with creation of a cosmetic urethrostomy has been performed in some cases to render them aesthetically acceptable to the owner and useful for performance activities.

Table 11-1
Laboratories Offering Animal Karyotyping Services

NAME	ADDRESS	CITY, STATE, ZIP	PHONE // WEB ADDRESS
Cytogenetics Laboratory	New Bolton Center 382 West Street Rd Uni of Pennsylvania	Kennett Square, PA 19348	215-444-5800 http://www.vet.upenn.edu/FacultyAndDepts/CSPHIL/MedicalGenetics/Services.cfm#cytogeneticsdef
Veterinary Cytogenetics Laboratory	Dept. Vet. Biology Rm 295 Animal Sci-Vet Med Bldg. 1988 Fitch Ave. Uni of Minnesota	St. Paul, MN 55106	612-624-3067 http://www.mvdl.umn.edu/
Genzyme Genetics	2000 Vivigen Way	Santa Fe, NM 87505	505-438-1111 http://www.genzymegenetics.com/aboutus/santa.htm
Veterinary Genetics Laboratory	School of Vet Med Uni of CA-Davis	Davis, CA 95616	916-752-2211 http://www.vgl.ucdavis.edu/default.htm

Gonadal Dysgenesis

✓ Sexual chromosome aneuploidy with karyotypes reported as 63X, 63X/64XX; and 63X/64XY.

✓ All breeds have been involved, but a greater incidence is reported in Arabians.

✓ Inbreeding is not reported to be a factor.

✓ This condition is not heritable and is not related to parental age.

✓ The human corollary is known as Turner's Syndrome (45X or 45XO).

✓ These animals have normal-appearing external female genitalia, small hypoplastic inactive ovaries, flaccid pre-pubertal uterus, flaccid cervix, endometrial hyoplasia, absent or irregular periods of estrous behavior, and may or may not show the characteristic short-coupled body stature, thick neck, and fat loin.

✓ Hormonal pattern is an elevated LH, very low estrogens, and very low progesterone.

✓ Diagnosis is by clinical exam, history, endocrinology, and karyotype. An endometrial biopsy will show atrophy of glandular structures (Figure 11-4).

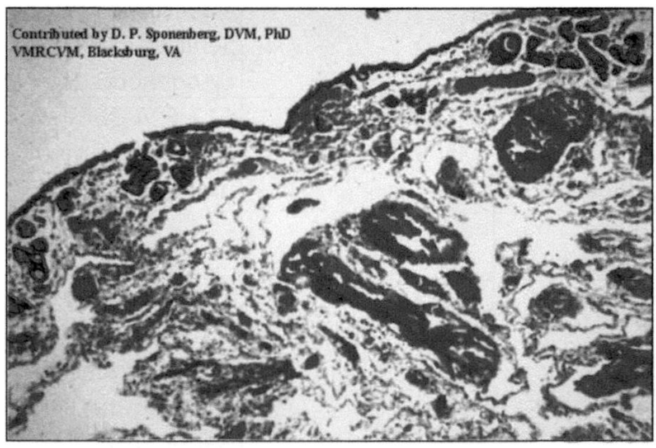

Figure 11-4 Histopathology of a mare's endometrium diagnosed with gonadal dysgenesis. There is almost complete atrophy of the normal endometrial structures.

Hybrids

✓ Normal donkey chromosome number is 62, 60 somatic chromosomes and 2 sex chromosomes. The jackass karyotype is 62XY and the jenny is 62XX.

✓ The hybrid offspring, mule (stallion x jenny) or hinny (jack x mare), chromosome number is either 63XY or 63XX.

✓ During gametogenesis in the hybrid offspring, marked irregularities occur in chromosome pairing before the first meiotic division at pachytene prophase; spermatogenesis is arrested in all males and oogenesis is inefficient in most females.

💣 Females may come into estrus, more rarely they may ovulate, but only a very few documented cases of pregnancy in the mule/hinny have been reported.

Ovarian Tumors and Conditions

The Merriam Webster Dictionary states that a tumor is any swollen or distended part; an abnormal, benign, or malignant mass of tissue that is not inflammatory, arises without obvious cause from cells of preexistent tissue, and possesses no physiologic function.

Granulosa-Theca Cell Tumor (GTCT)

✓ The most common ovarian tumor in the mare is the granulosa theca cell tumor (GTCT).

✓ GTCTs are hormonally active: the mare's behavior and clinical signs can be attributed to this.

✓ Mares with GTCT exhibit anestrous behavior in 5-10% of the total, nymphomania behavior in 5-8% of the total, and stallion-like behavior in about 50% of the total; behavior in the remainder is non-specific.

✓ Most affected mares are young to middle-aged (2-10 years of age).

✓ Suspect mares present with one large ovary usually with multiple cystic areas and loss of the ovulation fossa. The contralateral ovary is usually small, firm, and inactive.

✓ Some mares have been documented to have a GTCT which appeared as a unilocular or singlular cystic cavity. Others have been reported to have an active contralateral ovary.

✓ The affected ovary tends to have a characteristic appearance by ultrasonography but not all will have multiple hypoechoic areas indicative of small fluid pockets or cysts (Figures 11-5 and 11-6). ⊙

✓ Endocrine testing may reveal abnormally high serum testosterone (> 50-100 pg/ml), which is helpful in 50-60% of cases, low serum progesterone (< 1 ng/ml) in almost all affected mares, and elevated serum inhibin (> 0.7 ng/ml) in more than 90% of mares.

✓ Treatment is by unilateral ovariectomy.

✓ Following removal of the affected ovary, mares return to normal cyclicity/fertility in 3-12 mos.

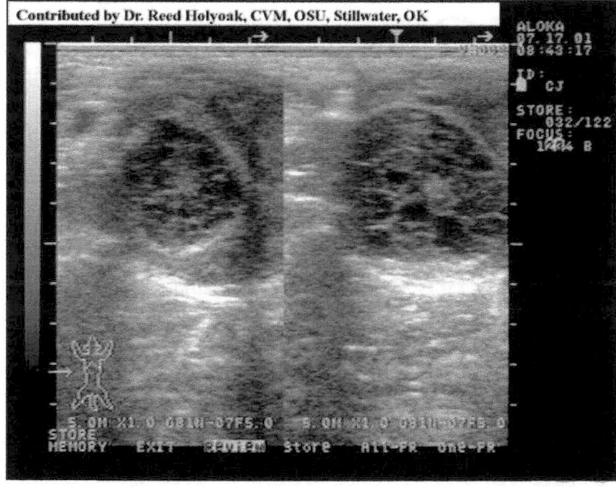

Figure 11-5
Ultrasonogram of a mare's ovary affected with granulosa theca cell tumor.

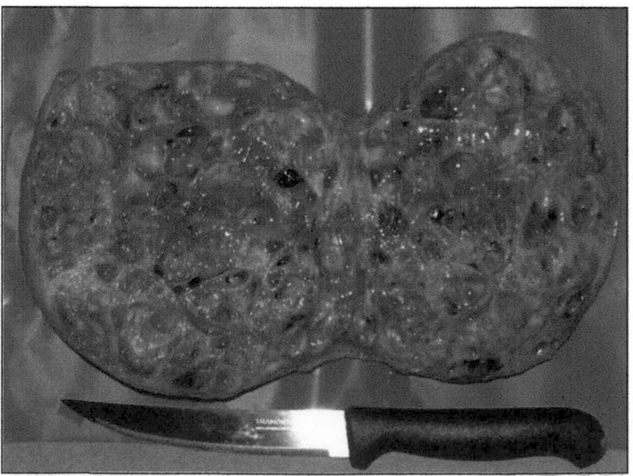

Figure 11-6
Cross-section of a mare's ovary affected by granulosa theca cell tumor.

Hematoma

✓ The most common cause of ovarian enlargement is an ovarian hematoma.

✓ These occasionally develop post-ovulation within the collapsed follicle, persisting for 1-3 estrous cycles with decreasing size over time.

✓ They constitute an excessively large corpus hemorrhagicum (CH).

✓ Differentiate from GTCT by ultrasonography, palpation of the opposite ovary, which is normal in size and activity, behavior, and time.

✓ No treatment is necessary. The mare will continue to cycle regularly from the opposite ovary and should conceive to ovulations from the non-affected side at the same rate as for an otherwise normal mare.

✓ Return to normal ovarian size and function is expected in most mares. Hematomas may occasionally obstruct the ovulation fossa and destroy the germinal epithelium making that ovary non-functional.

Cystadenoma (Primary Epithelial Origin Tumors)

✓ Tumor of the surface epithelium of the ovary. Most common unilaterally, but bilaterally affected ovaries have been reported.

✓ Tumors are benign, slow growing, and not hormonally active.

✓ Multiple to singular cystic areas within ovary on palpation or ultrasound which may appear very similar to GTCT.

✓ Serum testosterone usually ≤70 pg/ml, inhibin < 0.5 ng/ml, and progesterone > 1 ng/ml; contralateral ovary may be normal or small, firm, and inactive, rarely there will be bilaterally affected ovaries.

✓ Treatment may not be required as some mares will cycle and conceive, or consider ovariectomy.

Teratomas

✓ Benign, congenital tumors in young animals usually prepubertal and can be fast growing causing signs of abdominal enlargement and sometimes colic.

✓ Tumors may contain hair, pigment, and bone.

✓ Normal estrous cyclicity and even pregnancies have been reported in mares with ovarian teratoma.

✓ Treatment is by ovariectomy.

Lymphosarcoma

✓ Rarely encountered but potentially a cause of progressive cachexia and colic.

✓ Ovarian enlargement with metastasis have been noted along with neoplastic cells in cytologic samples recovered by abdominocentesis.

✓ Treatment is ineffective; ovariectomy is usually too late by the time a diagnosis is made to prevent metastasis.

Dysgerminoma

✓ Rare, malignant, and metastatic with a poor prognosis.

✓ Reported in some mares to be hormonally active.

✓ Hypertrophic osteodystrophy (HOD) associated with thoracic metastases.

✓ Treatment is by ovariectomy and you may need to consider chemotherapy to control growth and spread of metastases.

Arrhenoblastoma

✓ A rare hormonally-active ovarian tumor.

✓ Stallion-like behavior is usually associated with these tumors.

✓ Affected ovary is usually firm and smooth on palpation. The contralateral ovary is usually small and inactive.

✓ Serum testosterone is generally > 100 pg/ml and some have exceeded 2500 pg/ml.

✓ Treatment is by ovariectomy. Treated mares have returned to normal reproductive performance.

Cystic Ovaries

✓ The condition as recognized in dairy cows does not occur frequently in mares, but has been reported as a bilateral condition in at least one 6 year old mare.

🖐 The author has observed this condition in at least two other middle-aged mares, both affected bilaterally, that did not ovulate and would not conceive despite multiple attempts at breeding.

Paraovarian Cyst

✓ Paraovarian (tubal) cysts are not a direct cause of infertility unless the cyst happens to be closely associated with the oviduct and potentially cause occlusion or interference with the infundibulum's function during ovulation.

⊙ They are occasionally recognized on ultrasonography (Figure 11-7). They may also be observed directly by laparoscopy (Figure 11-8). See CD for demonstration of a laparoscopic view of a paraovarian cyst (Video 11-1).

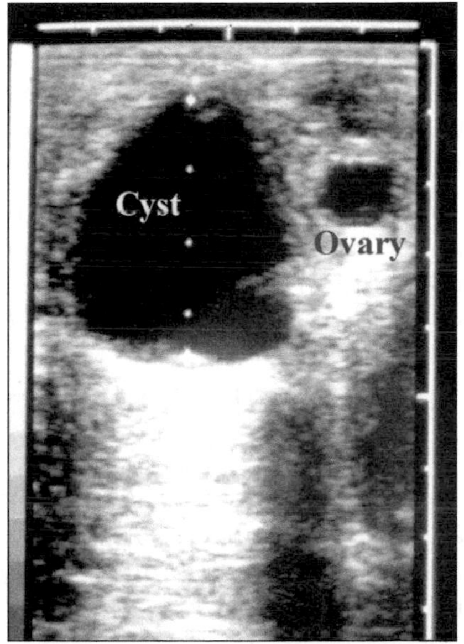

Figure 11-7
Ultrasonogram of a paraovarian cyst.

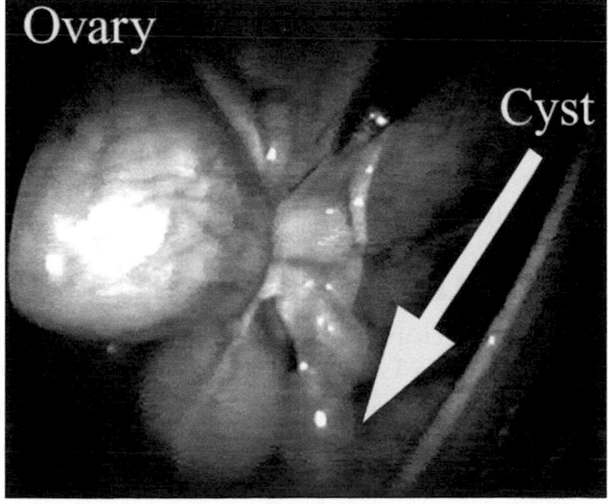

Figure 11-8
Laparoscopic view of a paraovarian cyst.

Other Causes of Non-Infectious Infertility

Twinning

✓ See Section 8, Management of Twin Conceptions.

✓ While it may seem incongruous to consider multiple embryos as a cause of infertility, the fact remains that many twins allowed to develop beyond 45-50 days of gestation will result in pregnancy wastage.

✓ More often than not, abortion of both twins occurs in mid- to late gestation, or a premature delivery of a weak or moribund surviving twin with one dead or mummified twin.

✓ Mares that abort due to twinning, or produce a weak or dead foal (or foals) are difficult to breed back and may suffer from retained fetal membranes in the immediate post-abortion or post-parturient period.

Early Embryonic Death

✓ See also Section 9.

✓ Barren mares have high fertilization rates equal to young maiden mares, but have low embryo recovery rates by embryo flushing at days 6-10 and have even lower pregnancy rates by ultrasound at day 14.

✓ Causes include:

Defective (chromosomal) embryo development (age-related)

Failure of oviductal transport

Abnormal uterine environment

✓ Embryo transfer studies have shown that the uterine environment in older barren mares is adequate to support embryos recovered from young donor mares.

Oviduct/Salpingitis

✓ See Section 6 for a review of the anatomy of the oviduct and Section 9 on Uterine Tube Considerations.

✓ One study on oviductal pathology reported that in 325 mares examined macroscopically and 124 examined microscopically, 88% had macroscopic lesions and 94% had microscopic lesions;

adhesions were the most frequent lesions observed and were most often bilateral.

✓ Salpingitis in the mare can be occlusive; inflammatory cell infiltrates of the oviductal epithelium narrow the lumen, but exudative secretions are infrequent. Regions of infundibulitis, isthmitis, and/or ampullitis occur.

✓ Ampullitis is more frequent than isthmitis and the right oviduct is more frequently affected than the left

✓ Diagnosis can be attempted by direct visualization using laparoscopy, direct visualization and catheterization for flushing by laparotomy, the starch granule test, a modified oviductal patency test using ultrasound-guided deposition of fluorescent microsphere beads, and by embryo recovery attempts.

Uterine Cysts/Lymphatic-Glandular Dilatations

✓ Uterine cysts are of one of two types: endometrial (glandular) or lymphatic.

✓ Endometrial cysts are typically smaller in dimension (1-10 mm) and are dispersed multifocally throughout one or more areas of the uterus. They result most commonly from chronic degenerative changes in the endometrium leading to periglandular fibrosis and glandular lumen restriction with dilatation of the glandular lumen resulting in its cystic distension.

✓ Lymphatic cysts are typically larger (>10 mm) and usually found in one to three locations. These result from lymphatic outflow stasis; surrounding endometrial tissues may have chronic inflammatory infiltrates or be normal histologically.

✓ Either condition requires use of ultrasonography or hysteroscopy for identification, but the larger lymphatic cysts may be identified by careful rectal palpation.

✓ Uterine cysts are degenerative and age-related changes.

✋ The relationship between the presence of cysts and fertility is still as yet unclear. They generally do not cause infertility by themselves except if large enough to obstruct embryo mobility during days 5-15.

✓ Many clinicians have observed normal embryonic development and pregnancy maintenance in the presence of one or more large uterine cysts.

Despite their potential for indicating significant underlying endometrial pathology, cysts may confuse the naïve diagnostician as well as the most experienced clinicians at the initial pregnancy diagnosis. Mistaking an embryo for a cyst and vice versa is a common challenge (Figures 11-9 and 11-10).

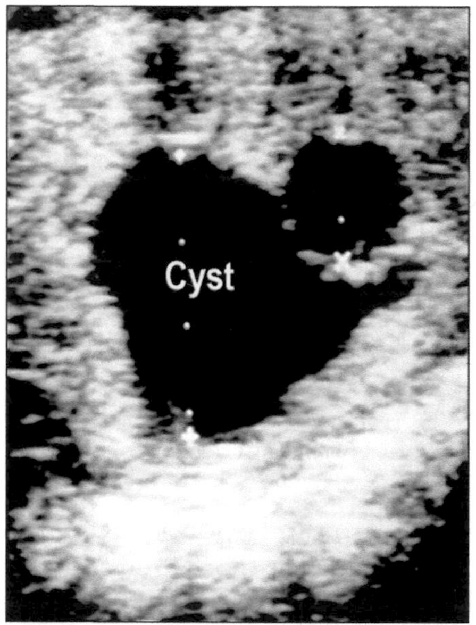

Figure 11-9 A large uterine cyst (left) next to a 14 day embryo (upper right) on uterine ultrasonography.

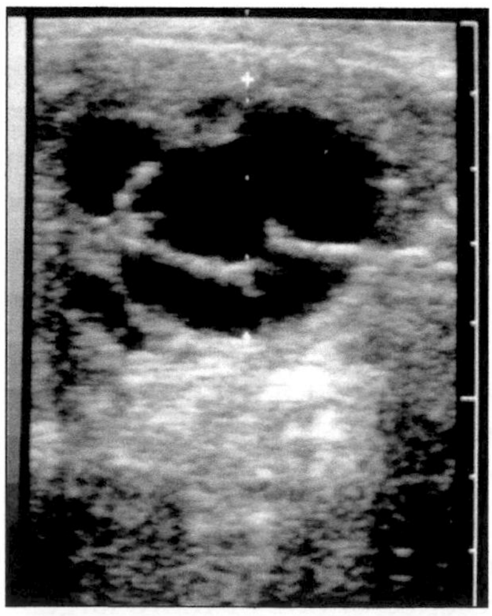

Figure 11-10 Multiple uterine cysts occluding the uterine lumen. This mare also had adhesions extending from one aspect of the endometrium to the opposite side.

✓ Most cysts are observed in older broodmares. One report found most cysts in 11 of 73 mares whose mean age was 13.4 years, whereas 62 of 73 mares without cysts were of a mean age of 6.9 years.

✓ A Swiss study in Thoroughbred mares reported that pregnancy rates at Days 14 and 40 were significantly ($P < 0.01$) lower in mares with cysts (77.6% and 71.4%) compared to mares without cysts (91.5% and 88.0%). This would suggest that the presence of uterine cysts may play an important role in the reduction of fertility. However, in this study when all mares were assigned to three age groups, < 7 years (n = 116), 7-14 years (n = 117) and > 14 years (n = 26), a significant ($P < 0.01$) increase in the number of endometrial cysts was observed with advancing age (4.3%, 29.1% and 73.1%, respectively). Is it age-related? Or cyst-related?

✓ Most clinicians will recommend breeding the mare with uterine cysts on one or more cycles in an attempt to see if she will carry her pregnancy in spite of them.

✓ It is prudent to record and map on a uterine chart the presence and size of all endometrial or lymphatic cysts identified prior to each attempted breeding.

✓ Cysts will appear and disappear occasionally throughout an estrous cycle, or between an ovulation and an initial pregnancy diagnosis at 14-15 days post-ovulation.

✓ In many mares with uterine cysts, there may also be intra-luminal adhesions present that cannot be detected by any means short of direct intrauterine palpation or visualization by hysteroscopy.

✓ Treatment options have included electrocoagulation, laser ablation, direct puncture by endometrial biopsy forceps, manual rupture, and various intrauterine infusions with saline, warm (40-45°C) hypertonic saline, and magnesium sulfate.

☞ In this author's opinion, cysts that are significantly large (i.e., > 20 mm) warrant treatment by hysteroscopic neodymium:ytrium aluminum garnet (Nd:YAG) laser ablation.

Uterine Tumors/Neoplasia

✓ Hematoma is the most commonly occurring tumor of the uterus or its associated structures. They generally occur along the vaginal wall, but may also involve the cervix, and extend to, or originate in, the endometrium, myometrium, or broad ligament of the uterus. They can be focal and spherical (10-20 cm diameter) or extensive and oblong obstructing most of the pelvic inlet.

💣 Hematoma formation in the broad ligament can be life-threatening if the hemorrhage is not confined by the mesometrial tissues.

✓ Hematoma are usually self-limiting if the hemorrhage is controlled. They may secondarily become infected and an abscess develop which may require drainage and lavage per vaginum.

✓ Leiomyoma is a smooth muscle tumor which typically has a very firm varied size polymorphic feel on palpation per rectum or per vaginum. Diagnosis is made by biopsy and histopathology. Treatment is by sharp resection or laser ablation if it can be performed without jeopardizing the integrity of the cervix.

✓ Endometrial adenocarcinoma has been reported. The mare was presented with signs of depression, anorexia, weight loss, ventral edema, and abdominal distension of 5 weeks duration. Transrectal ultrasonography revealed numerous hyperechoic nodules (3-20 mm diameter) distributed throughout the pelvic canal, uterus, broad ligament, and intestinal serosa. Abdominocentesis revealed a copious modified transudate without evidence of neoplasia.

Abnormalities of the Cervix

✓ Traumatic or foaling injury adhesions or scars; cervicitis leading to adhesions.

✓ Tumors (leiomyomas).

✓ Cervical atony due to anestrus, age, or poor body condition

✓ Congenital incompetency and aplasia have been reported.

✓ Repair of cervical lacerations can be performed using a single layer closure technique 2-3 days after AI and ovulation.

Autoantibodies to Zona Pellucida

✓ Out of 65 infertile mares, 7 had serum antibody titers reactive to porcine zona pellucida (ZP) antigens as detected by an indirect immunofluorescence method.

✓ In other species, antibodies develop against ZP and effectively block sperm receptor sites at zona surface.

✓ Also antibodies against ZP have prevented hatching of fertilized embryos.

✓ Multiple sampling may be necessary to eliminate false negative results in testing.

✓ Treatment may be attempted with prednisolone or other corticosteroid therapy.

Sperm Agglutinins/Equine Anti-Sperm Antibodies (ASA)

✓ Mares known to have positive serum titers to equine ASA inseminated with equine semen have lower pregnancy rates than mares that have negative serum equine ASA titers.

✓ ASA reduce conception by interfering with sperm transport by binding to sperm surfaces and decreasing motility.

✓ Many sperm bound by ASA have increased phagocytosis rates by uterine-derived PMN leukocytes and decreased survival in vivo.

✓ ASA have also been shown to block sperm attachment to oviductal epithelium as well as to the surface of the oocyte's zona pellucida.

✓ ASA in rabbits and humans have been shown to reduce embryo survival rates once conception has occurred.

✓ ASA have been documented to occur in stallions with decreased reproductive efficiency or subfertility.

✓ ASA titers in the mare can be obtained using a specific equine ELISA.

✓ ASA in the stallion have been controlled or diminished by corticosteroid therapy during the breeding season, returning the affected males to near normal conception rates.

Hypothyroidism

✓ The role of equine hypothyroidism in equine reproductive performance remains controversial.

✓ Sole reliance on serum thyroxine (T4) levels as a means of diagnosing hypothyroidism is suspect at best in diagnostic accuracy.

✓ In one recent study of 329 mares, there was no direct relationship between serum T4 levels and pregnancy ($p=0.282$). There was also no significant relationship found between thyroid hormone supplementation and pregnancy at 15-16 days post-ovulation.

Equine Cushing's Disease (ECD)

✓ The relationship between ECD and infertility in the mare remains unclear. Some mares with ECD are able to conceive and deliver normal foals and others have difficulty conceiving.

✓ Most horses affected with ECD are older at an average age of 20 years. Thus it remains to be seen if the infertility is age- or ECD-related.

✓ ECD results from an excessive secretion of pro-opiomelanocortin (POMC) derived from peptides from the pituitary pars intermedia (PI). The PI does not have a negative feedback response to cortisol and does not respond to corticotropin-releasing hormone.

✓ A Peripheral Cushing's Syndrome has been reported in which it is believed that an altered cortisol metabolism at the cellular level produces signs consistent with ECD, such as obesity and laminitis.

✓ Signs of ECD include hirsutism, obesity, thick cresty neck, lethargy, hyperhydrosis, tachypnea, polyuria/polydipsia, immunosuppression, and laminitis. Not every horse affected with ECD will have each or any combination of these signs.

✓ Clinical laboratory findings may include hyperglycemia, elevated hepatic enzymes, neutrophilia, lymphopenia, and anemia.

✓ The dexamethasone suppression test is the preferred diagnostic modality to confirm suspected cases of ECD. A blood sample is obtained prior to starting the test. Forty µg of dexamethasone/kg of body weight are given by intramuscular injection between 4 and 6 p.m. A second blood sample is obtained about 19 hours later, between 10 a.m. and noon the following day. The samples are submitted for plasma cortisol. Cortisol levels > 10 ng/ml in the post-dexamethasone sample are diagnostic of ECD.

✓ Pergolide is an effective treatment for ECD at an initial dose of 1 mg/ 450kg PO q24h. Pergolide is a dopamine agonist and may suppress mammary development in late term pregnant mares. They should have pergolide therapy discontinued starting 30 days prior to their expected foaling date.

✓ Cyproheptadine, a serotonin antagonist, has also been used as an alternate therapy for ECD therapy. It is administered at 0.25 mg/kg PO q12-24h.

Nutrition and Body Condition

✓ See Section 3, Preventive Medicine Program for Broodmares, Nutrition.

Breeding Mismanagement

✓ See Section 7, Breeding Management.

Transitional Season

✔ During the transition from winter anestrous to spring polyestrous, many mares show behavioral signs of estrus without corresponding follicular development. Many such mares are bred based on these signs of heat. When they fail to conceive many owners/farm managers consider them to be infertile. This is a simple mismanagement problem, which can have counterproductive consequences, especially for older barren mares.

✔ Treatment options are discussed in Section 5.

Prolonged Lifespan of CL

✔ Prolonged diestrus is a common estrous cycle abnormality. Farm managers or mare owners who fail to use a means of positive pregnancy diagnosis (e.g., transrectal ultrasonography) may consider mares that fail to return to heat as pregnant, later discovering them to be barren and thus an infertile or problem mare.

✔ Diagnosis is by close veterinary examination using ultrasonography to view the ovaries and evidence of structure(s) consistent with a corpus luteum or corpora lutea (see Figure 6-5). Alternatively a blood sample may be obtained and the mare's plasma progesterone measured for evidence of an active CL (see Table 8-2).

✔ Treatment options are found in Table 5-1 using PGF2-a.

Environmental Stress

✔ Transportation, confinement, extremes in temperature, and social interaction / separation have all been reported to be stressors of domestic animals inducing failure to exhibit estrous cycle activity, silent heats, and pregnancy wastage.

✔ Transportation stress in early pregnant mares has been studied and did reveal elevation of plasma cortisol and decrease in progesterone levels, but did not show increased incidence of early embryonic or fetal loss.

✔ Cold inclement weather stress may inhibit mares from showing overt signs of estrus especially early in the breeding season and may delay or prolong the period of follicular growth prior to ovulation.

✔ Heat stress and high humidity are associated with some mares entering into a period of estrous cycle inactivity or quiescence as well as with occasional prolongation of the lifespan of the CL. Whether the latter is simply a seasonal effect or truly associated with heat stress remains to be determined, as both tend to occur at the same time of the year (i.e., mid to late summer).

Pregnancy

✓ In breeding management systems where mares are bred individually and good records are maintained it is unlikely that pregnant mares would be presented as infertility cases. However, in cases where records are poor to nonexistent, or mistakes have been made in the identity of the mare, or misdiagnosis of pregnancy status has occurred, it is prudent to make certain that a mare presented for failing to cycle or show signs of estrus or otherwise as infertile is not ALREADY pregnant!

✓ See Section 8, Pregnancy Diagnosis.

Section 12

Assisted Reproductive Technologies

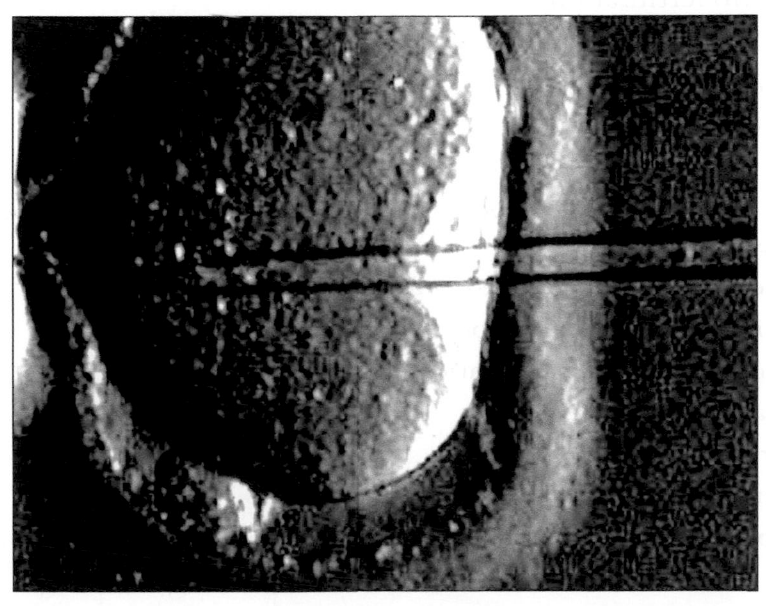

New techniques to assist reproduction have placed a considerable burden on the scientific and veterinary medical communities. Practitioners must not only be familiar with the indications for each of the techniques available, but must also be able to balance between the benefits and the risks from each procedure for their clients. We as a profession must also ensure that all these techniques are ethically sound and have as their sole purpose the improvement of animal reproductive efficiency.

Components of Assisted Reproductive Technologies

Assisted reproductive technologies (ART) include several procedures employed to bring about conception without mating. They include, but are not limited to the following:

Artificial insemination / intrauterine insemination

Embryo recovery, transfer, and cryopreservation

Gamete intrafallopian transfer

Intrafollicular transfer of oocyte(s)

Intracytoplasmic sperm injection

In vitro fertilization

Oocyte retrieval, transfer, and cryopreservation

Tubal embryo transfer

Xenogeneic gamete intrafallopian transfer

Zygote intrafallopian transfer

The technologies involved in performing many of these procedures include:

Superovulation/controlled ovarian hyperstimulation

Follicular aspiration of oocyte/oocyte maturation in vitro

Sperm collection/capacitation/cryopreservation

Laparoscopy

Ultrasonography

Micromanipulation of gametes and zygotes

Embryo culturing, sexing, and cryopreservation

The Realities of ART

✓ It is not likely that the rate of establishing a pregnancy from each egg by IVF or ICSI followed by embryo transfer can improve on the normal rate of reproductive efficiency.

✓ The theoretical maximum success per egg (oocyte) retrieved in any one estrous cycle is likely to be in the 20 to 30% range. Most are lower!

Why ART in Horses?

The reproductive efficiency of mares and stallions decreases with age.

Potential value of the expected progeny.

Value of one parent in another occupation.

Uterine tube (Fallopian tube, oviduct) blockage.

Hostile uterine environment (endometrosis, chronic degenerative endometritis)

Male factor infertility or low sperm numbers in the stallion.

Limits Imposed

Limits may be imposed by

✓ Lack of success to date in superovulation of the mare (average is 3 ova per mare). This is attributable to the relatively limited area available in the mare's ovulation fossa for ovulation to occur in and to the relatively large size of each follicle prior to ovulation.

✓ Age of the individual female providing the oocyte (Table 12-1).

✓ Poor success in cryopreservation of embryos.

✓ Inconsistencies in oocyte maturation protocols.

✓ Lack of understanding of stallion sperm capacitation.

✓ Breed registry regulations.

✓ Costs of procedures.

Table 12-1
Pregnancy Success Rates Using ART Versus Age of the Oocyte Donor

Parameter measured in 1997	Age of oocyte donor (yrs) < 35	35-37	38-40	> 40
Number of cycles	24,581	12,733	10,997	6,691
Pregnancies per 100 cycles	35.7	31.3	22.8	13.2
Live births per 100 transfers	35.9	31.4	22.5	10.9
Live births per 100 cycles	30.7	25.5	17.1	7.6

Parameter measured in 1999	Age of oocyte donor (yrs) < 35	35-37	38-40	> 40
Number of cycles	29,682	15,291	12,848	5,302
Pregnancies per 100 cycles	37.3	31.6	24.4	15.9
Live births per 100 transfers	32.2	26.2	18.5	9.7
Live births per 100 cycles	37.8	32.4	24.2	13.6

From: http://www.cdc.gov/nccdphp/drh/art.htm

Artificial Insemination (AI) and Intrauterine Insemination (IUI)

✓ This is a relatively low tech ART which deposits sperm directly into the uterus by-passing the vagina and cervix.

✓ AI is a predecessor to the IUI procedure used in women.

✓ Low-dose sperm deposition using hysteroscopy, or deep intrauterine insemination at, or on, the uterine-tubal junction (UTJ; papilla of the oviductal sphincter as it communicates with uterus at the tip of each uterine horn) is a newer method of AI in the mare. Recent studies have demonstrated acceptable conception rates using as few as 5 million sperm per mare (optimum numbers for typical transcervical AI range from 100-500 million sperm per mare).

✓ See also Section 5, Breeding Management.

Embryo Transfer (ET)

✓ Embryo transfer is the most widely used ART in the mare.

✓ The reasons for the commercial application of ET in the mare include:

- Acquiring foals from reproductively unserviceable mares
- Acquiring multiple foals from individual donor mares each year
- Acquiring foals from donor mares during their athletic performance years
- Acquiring foals from junior or young maiden mares
- Acquiring foals from mares with other health problems (e.g., chronic laminitis, fractured pelvis)

✓ There are two physiological peculiarities of the mare which place limitations on equine ET which are not present in other domestic species. The first is that mares cannot be successfully superovulated at this time. The second is the variation in length of the mare's estrous cycle. Neither the onset of estrus, nor its end, provide a reliable indication of time of ovulation.

✓ The first successful equine embryo transfer was reported in 1972.

✓ A technique for cooling equine embryos has been developed, which is a practical method of short-term (up to 24 hr) storage and transportation. This allows the embryo to be collected on the farm and shipped to a distant facility for transfer to a suitable recipient mare. The ability to transport cooled embryos provides practitioners with the opportunity to offer embryo transfer services without the need to maintain their own recipient mare band.

✓ The donor mare and recipient mares should be examined thoroughly prior to their use (See Section 6, Breeding Serviceability Exam). If abnormalities are identified in the donor mare that warrant treatment (e.g., bacterial or mycotic endometritis), appropriate therapy should be initiated before embryo transfer procedures are performed.

✓ Selection and management of recipient mares is an equally important aspect that will affect the success of an equine ET program. Recipient mares should have normal estrous cycles and be free of uterine and/or ovarian abnormalities. Their optimum age should be between 3 to 10 years.

✓ Synchronizing estrus between donor and recipient mares can be accomplished with routine protocols using PGF2a alone or in combination with exogenous progesterone (See Section 5, Seasonality, the Estrous Cycle, and its Manipulation and Artificial Control).

✓ The window of opportunity for synchrony between ovulations in recipient and donor mares is plus 1 to minus 3 days; the recipient mare(s) can ovulate 1 day prior to and up to 3 days after the donor mare.

✓ The donor mare should be monitored according to good breeding management techniques as described in Section 7, Breeding Management. Use appropriate methods to assist ovulation (hCG or deslorelin) to enhance chances of conception. While embryo recoveries have been successfully performed from donor mares bred with frozen, transported, or fresh semen, the best success is with the use of fresh semen.

✓ Embryos are selectively transported through the oviduct into the uterus on day 5 to 6 post-ovulation at which time they are at the compact morula to early blastocyst stage of development (Figures 12-1 and 12-2) ⊙. After entering the uterine lumen, the size of the embryo increases dramatically as it develops into an expanded blastocyst (Figure 12-3). ⊙

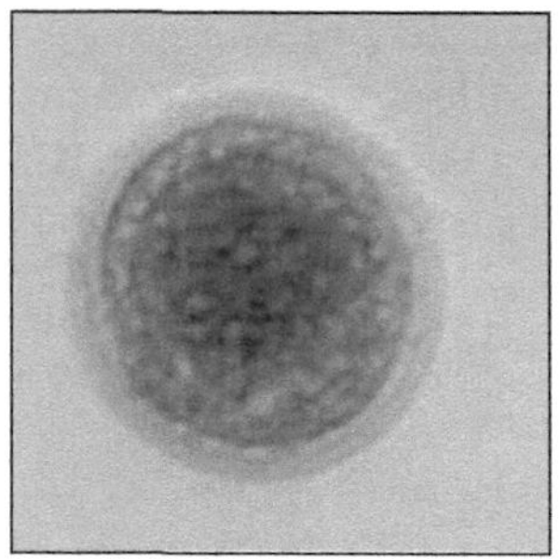

Figure 12-1
Equine morula.

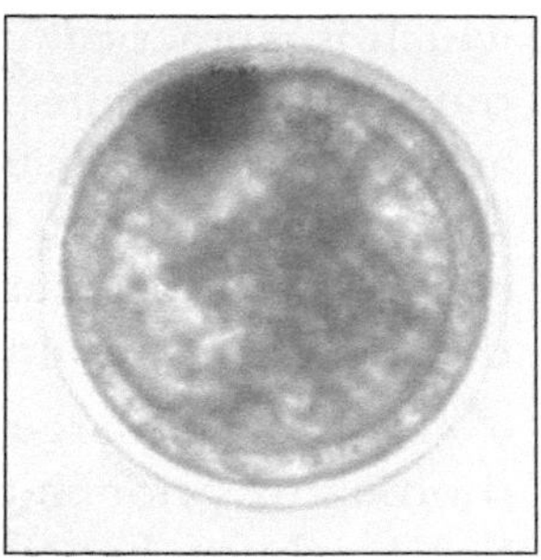

Figure 12-2
Equine blastocyst.

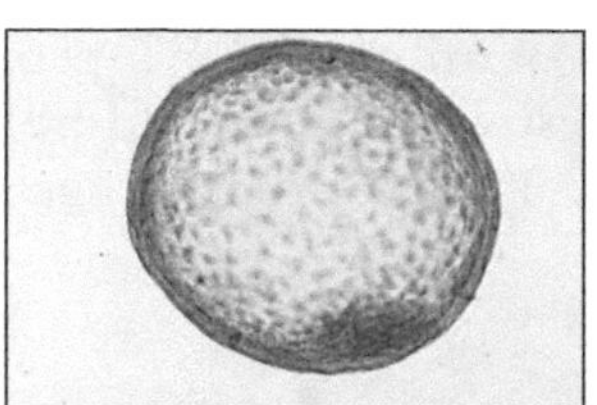

Figure 12-3 Equine expanded blastocyst.

✓ Although embryos can be recovered over the range of days 6 to 9, the optimal time of embryo collection is day 7 or 8 post-ovulation.

✓ Although embryo transfer was initially proposed as a promising method for obtaining foals from aged subfertile mares, experiments utilizing oocyte transfer and embryo transfer have documented that many oocytes/embryos produced by aged subfertile mares are inherently defective. Embryos from such mares have low survival rates after transfer to recipient mares; therefore, aged subfertile mares are not optimal donor candidates for embryo transfer (Figures 12-4 and 12-5).

✓ See also Section 9, Early Embryonic Loss.

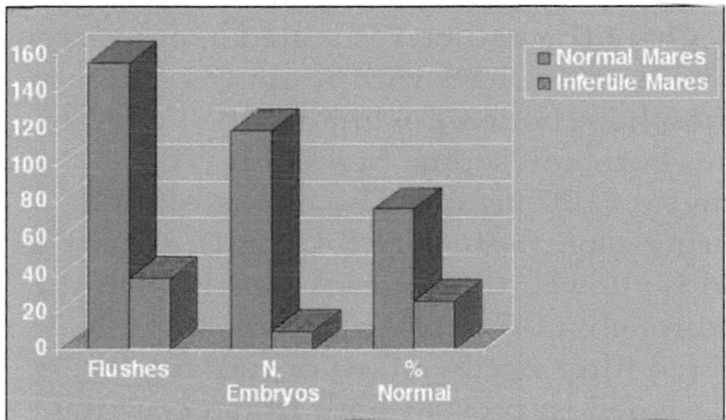

Figure 12-4 Embryo transfer in mares, number of flush attempts, the number of normal embryos recovered, and the percent of normal embryos recovered between normal young mares and older infertile mares. (From Imel, et al: JAVMA, 1981 179 (10):987.)

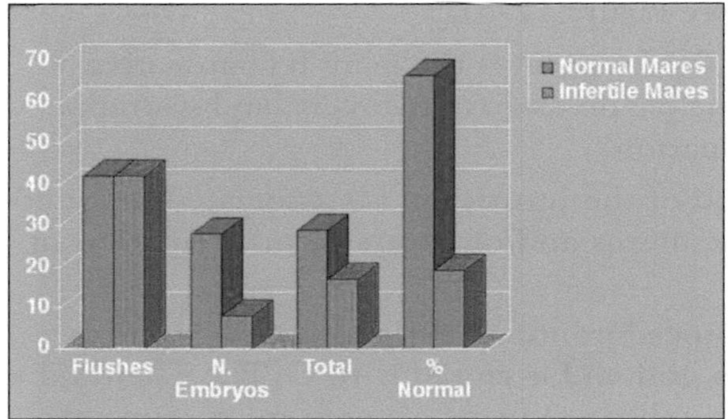

Figure 12-5 Embryo transfer in mares. Embryo transfer in mares, an equal number of flush attempts, the number of normal embryos recovered, the percent of all embryos recovered, and the percent of normal embryos recovered between normal young mares and older infertile mares. (From Woods, et al: Cornell Vet, 1986, 76(4):386.)

Embryo Flushing Procedure

✓ The procedure for embryo flushing is very similar to the uterine lavage technique described in Section 10.

✓ The mare is restrained in stocks, and her perineal area is cleansed with a mild detergent, rinsed thoroughly with clean water and dried. The operator then places a sterile plastic sleeve over his or her arm, applies sterile lubricant, and introduces a sterile balloon-tipped, 80 cm silicone catheter that has an inside diameter of 8.0 mm (33Fr)(see Figure 10-7). After entering the vagina, the catheter is passed through the cervix into the uterine body, and the balloon cuff is inflated with approximately 80 ml sterile saline. The balloon is positioned back against the cervix to prevent loss of fluid. Once the catheter is seated appropriately, the uterus is flushed three to four times with warm (37.5°C) modified Dulbecco's phosphate buffered saline (DPBS) containing 1% (v/v) fetal or newborn calf serum, penicillin (100 units/ml), and streptomycin (100 µg/ml). The uterus is filled with 1-2 L of DPBS during each flush (3 to 8 L total). After filling the uterus, the fluid is allowed to flow back out through the catheter and is passed through a 0.75-0.80 µ embryo filter. It is important that the embryo filter not overflow or run dry; filters are available that are designed to prevent both from occurring. The fluid passing through the filter is collected to monitor its recovery. Before the final flush, the uterus is massaged per rectum, to aid suspension of the embryo(s) in the medium and enhance fluid recovery. The majority (>90%) of fluid infused into the uterus should be recovered, and it should be free of cellular debris or blood (see Figure 12-6).

✓ Recovery of cloudy fluid indicates the mare had an active endometritis at the time of the embryo recovery, and warrants further diagnostic evaluation.

✓ Blood contamination of the return fluid is associated with too vigorous massage of the uterus and/or excessive manipulation of the catheter.

✓ After the flushing procedure, the filter cup is emptied into a sterile search dish with grid and is rinsed with DPBS. The fluid is then examined for the embryo(s) using a stereo-microscope at 10-20x magnification. Large embryos (~ Day 8) are often visible with the naked eye.

✓ When an embryo(s) is identified, it is "washed" by transferring it sequentially through at least three 1 ml wells of DPBS with

10% (v/v) serum that has been filtered through a 0.22 µ syringe-filter; after "washing" the embryo is placed into a small Petri dish (35 x 10 mm) containing the same medium.

✓ The embryo is then examined at high magnification (40 to 80x) and graded on a scale of 1 (excellent) to 4 (poor).

✓ Embryos can be handled using a 0.25 or 0.5 ml semen-freezing straw or 25 µL glass capillary pipette attached to an appropriate syringe. Anytime an embryo is drawn into a handling instrument, the medium containing the embryo should be surrounded on each side by an air bubble and fluid medium. This prevents the embryo from accidentally being wicked out of the instrument should the tip touch something absorbent. The process of picking up and depositing an embryo should be observed under the microscope.

✓ Transfer of the embryo should take place as soon as possible after collection, as it has been shown that pregnancy rates drop dramatically if the embryo is out of the mare for more than 1-2 hours. The transfer can be made either surgically or non-surgically.

✓ In the surgical approach, it can either be a midline approach under general anesthesia, or by a standing flank approach under mild sedation and local anesthesia. Pregnancy rates of 75-80% can be achieved.

✓ Non-surgical transfer (transcervical) is easy to perform. However pregnancy rates are not as high (60-70%), and success is more dependent upon the skill of the operator than the technique involved. It should be performed smoothly and rapidly, using a technique similar to a routine AI.

✓ Non-surgical embryo transfer can been performed using a standard AI pipette, a single-use sterile insemination gun, or a reusable stainless steel insemination gun with a sterile protective sheath.

✓ A newer approach for embryo transfer using transvaginal ultrasound-guided intrauterine injection of the embryo has recently been described. The initial data indicate a 78% successful transfer rate in establishment of pregnancy (18 pregnancies out of 23 embryos transferred).

✓ An example timetable for embryo transfer is presented in Table 12-2.

Table 12-2
Example Timetable for Equine Embryo Transfer

DAY OR TIME	PROCEDURE
DAY 0	$PGF_2\alpha$ (5mg) to donor and recipients
DAY 13	$PGF_2\alpha$ (5mg) to donor and recipients
DAY 16	Beginning of estrus
DAY 17	Palpation and ultrasound of donor and recipients. Monitor follicle size and ovulation. BREED DONOR or give 3,000 IU of hCG IV to donor and recipients when follicle size is appropriate.
DAY 18	Palpation and ultrasound of donor and recipients. Monitor follicle size and ovulation. Breed donor if she was not bred 24h previously.
DAY 19	Palpation and ultrasound of donor and recipients. Monitor follicle size and ovulation.
DAY 20	Palpation and ultrasound of donor and recipients. Monitor follicle size and ovulation. Breed donor if she was not bred 24h previously.
DAY 21	Palpation and ultrasound of donor and recipients. Monitor follicle size and ovulation.
OVULATION (Day 0)	**Noted in donor and recipients**
DAY +7 to +8	Embryo flush procedure. Embryo transfer procedure IF a good quality embryo is recovered. $PGF_2\alpha$ to donor and to recipients IF no embryo was recovered.
DAY +14 to +16	PREGNANCY EXAM – Rectal palpation & ultrasound.
DAY +21 to +28	PREGNANCY CHECK - Rectal palpation & ultrasound.
DAY +45	Final PREGNANCY CHECK - Rectal palpation & ultrasound.

Embryo Shipment

✓ While awaiting packaging for transport, equine embryos are tolerant of temperatures between room temperature (25°C) and body temperature (37°C). Efforts should be made to prevent rapid or extreme changes in temperature.

✓ Equine embryos are cooled and transported using nutrient media such as Ham's F-10. Prior to its use, Ham's F-10 medium must be buffered by diffusing a mixture of 90% N2, 5% O_2, and 5% CO_2 gas through the medium for 3-5 minutes, after which it is supplemented with 10% (v/v) fetal or newborn calf serum, penicillin (100 units/ml), and streptomycin (100 µg/ml).

✓ Because Ham's F-10 medium must be "gassed" prior to use, it requires an appropriate compressed gas cylinder and regulator; therefore, many practitioners choose to have the embryo transfer facility that will receive the embryo provide Ham's F-10 as part of an embryo shipping kit.

⊙ Emcare™ Embryo Holding Solution has recently been shown to be a suitable alternative to Ham's F10 as an embryo shipping medium. It requires no advanced preparation. (http://homepages.ihug.co.nz/~icpltd/emcare.htm)

✓ To package the embryo for shipment, the nutrient medium is filter-sterilized (0.22 µ syringe filter) into a 5 ml snap-cap tube, leaving a small air gap at the top of the tube. The embryo is then carefully transferred into the medium, the cap is securely snapped onto the tube, and the tube is wrapped with Parafilm®. A 50-ml centrifuge tube is then filled with medium (unfiltered), and the 5-ml tube containing the embryo is placed into the 50-ml centrifuge tube. The cap of the 50-ml centrifuge tube is closed eliminating as much air as possible, and it is wrapped with Parafilm®.

✓ The packaged embryo is then placed into an Equitainer® (see Figure 2-4). This passively cools the embryo to 5°C. Using this system, embryos can remain viable for at least 24 hours, during which time they can be transported via commercial airline or priority overnight delivery to the facility where recipient mares have been prepared for the transfer.

Embryo Cryopreservation

Background

✓ Mammalian embryos have been successfully frozen and stored since 1972 when live mice where obtained after the transfer of freeze-thawed morulae. In humans, the first birth from a frozen embryo occurred in 1984 in Australia. This cryotechnology, derived from rodent and cattle routines, became a necessary part of IVF programs in order to avoid the risks of multiple pregnancies following the transfer of large numbers of embryos. At present, embryo freezing is a widespread, routine procedure in human infertility clinics.

Indications

To preserve multiple embryos where immediate transfer is not desired

To avoid synchronization problems between donor and recipients

To maintain embryos enabling their international shipment

Usual Procedure

✓ Human embryos can be successfully cryopreserved by protocols using 1,2 propanediol (PROH), dimethylsulfoxide (DMSO) or glycerol. Each of these cryoprotectants gives an optimal result when used at a particular embryo developmental stage : PROH or DMSO for zygotes or cleaved embryos, glycerol for blastocysts. No definite conclusions can be made regarding which embryonic stage is the best to preserve, from zygote to blastocyst. Embryos of lesser quality can be successfully frozen, but the best survival rates are obtained with embryos displaying the best morphology. Straws or ampules used for freezing embryos should be carefully and permanently labeled for identification purposes. After thawing, only embryos containing at least half of the initial number of blastomeres within an intact zona pellucida have optimal viability. The length of storage might be extended to at least 5 years without any impairment in embryonic viability as reported by retrospective studies.

✓ Freezing of equine embryos is not as simple as in the bovine, probably due to the fairly high lipid content of equine embryos and their relatively large size. Best results for freezing have been achieved using early to late morula stages obtained by surgical oviductal flushes.

✓ Cryopreservation of small equine embryos (< 300 μ) has been more successful than with larger embryos (300-1100 μ). It is postulated that the thickness of the larger equine embryo's capsule interferes with cryoprotectant permeability.

✓ Pretreating collected day 7 or 8 equine embryos with trypsin (0.2%, w:v) for 15 minutes prior to a standard method of cryopreservation, in one recent study improved post-thaw embryo survival and pregnancy rate in large (> 1000 μ) transferred embryos (3 of 11 were successful).

Gamete Intrafallopian Transfer (GIFT)

Background

✓ GIFT is an ART developed in 1984 by infertility specialists at the University of Texas Health Science Center, San Antonio, TX. The GIFT procedure allows fertilization to occur just as it does during naturally occurring matings.

Usual Procedure

✓ Male gametes (sperm) and female gametes (ova or eggs) are placed separately into a catheter and deposited into the recipient's uterine (Fallopian) tube during a surgical procedure (laparoscopy or laparotomy). Ultrasound is used to retrieve donor oocytes through the flank or through the anterior vaginal wall. Sperm can be fresh, transported, or frozen and thawed. Sperm preparation procedures such as a "wash" or a swim-up procedure using Percoll are usually performed prior to mixing sperm with the ova and the GIFT procedure.

Advantages of the GIFT Procedure

✓ The higher success rates reported with the GIFT technique (compared to IVF) is related to the fact that GIFT relies on the body's own natural processes and timetable to produce a healthy environment for fertilization, and early embryo development. GIFT offers a number of distinct advantages over other infertility treatments:

> Male factors: males with low sperm numbers or poor sperm function may be able to achieve conceptions using this method

Female factors: many of the same for ET above, but more specific for females with damage to or blockage of only one Fallopian tube, and damage to the cervix, where ET would be less optimal.

Immunological factors; antibodies present on either the sperm or in the uterus that may prevent sperm from reaching or fertilizing the eggs

GIFT in the Horse

✓ In vivo matured oocyte(s) obtained by transvaginal ultrasound-guided follicular aspiration from the donor's ovary, followed by surgical transfer of oocyte(s) to a recipient mare's oviduct in a solution mixed with sperm from the stallion. The recipient's own follicle does not need to be removed or aspirated as the donated gametes are placed in the opposite oviduct, and the likelihood of fertilization of her own oocyte is extremely small. The recipient may also have the opposite oviduct ligated to prevent her own ovum from being fertilized.

✓ Other than the ability to produce a follicle with a viable oocyte, there are few other qualifications for the donor.

✓ The recipient must be as reproductively fit as possible to maximize success of the procedure. She should have a good frame size to allow ready access to her ovary/oviduct through standing flank laparotomy, and preferably not be a maiden. Maiden mares frequently do not have sufficient broad ligament laxity to allow easy access to the oviduct through a standing flank approach for the GIFT procedure.

✓ 70% success with in vitro matured oocytes from normal young mares.

✓ 30% success with similarly treated oocytes from older barren mares.

✓ GIFT success with fresh semen from fertile stallions has ranged from 27 to 82%.

✓ GIFT success rates using semen from transported-cooled or frozen-thawed sources has been comparably less than with that of freshly collected stallion semen.

Intracytoplasmic Sperm Injection (ICSI)

Background

✓ In the last two decades, in-vitro fertilization (IVF) has been successful in the treatment of long-standing infertility due to tubal disease, idiopathic and male-factor infertility. It is well documented that the results of IVF in male infertility cases are not as good as those in men with normal semen parameters. In andrological infertility, only 20-30% of the inseminated cumulus-oocyte complexes are normally fertilized, which is much lower than the 60-70% fertilization rate in patients with tubal infertility. Absence of fertilization may occur in about one third of the cycles. It has been the experience of all centers for reproductive medicine that a certain number of patients with andrological infertility cannot be helped by standard IVF treatment. Furthermore, a sizable number of couples cannot be accepted for IVF if the number of progressively motile spermatozoa with normal morphology available for insemination is below a certain threshold number such as 500,000 (human). In the past decade, assisted fertilization procedures have been developed to circumvent the barriers that prevent sperm access to the ooplasma, namely the zona pellucida and the ooplasmic membrane. Successful fertilization, embryo development, pregnancies and births have been reported after partial zona dissection (PZD) and subzonal insemination (SUZI). In 1992, the first pregnancies and births were obtained by intracytoplasmic sperm injection (ICSI). The results of several hundreds of cycles of assisted fertilization by SUZI and ICSI, and a controlled comparison of ICSI and SUZI on sibling oocytes, indicated that the normal fertilization rate after ICSI is substantially higher than after SUZI. The higher fertilization rate and similar cleavage rate resulted in more embryos for transfer after ICSI, and high implantation rates have been obtained. Many human infertility clinics have adopted ICSI as the sole procedure of assisted fertilization.

✓ ICSI was performed in 751 couples, accounting for 987 menstrual cycles, between 1993 and 1995 at the Center for Reproductive Medicine and Infertility at The New York Hospital, Cornell Medical Center. The 987 cycles of ICSI resulted in 943 embryo transfer procedures; 547 (55%) achieved a biochemical pregnancy, and 437 (44%) resulted in a clinical pregnancy. There were four ectopic pregnancies, and 51 miscarriages or abortions. The delivery rate per cycle was 39%.

Advantages

✓ ICSI can be carried out with fresh or frozen-thawed ejaculated spermatozoa, with fresh and frozen-thawed epididymal spermatozoa, and with spermatozoa isolated from a shredded testicular biopsy.

Indications for ICSI with Ejaculated Spermatozoa

✓ Severe male-factor infertility and fertilization failure after standard IVF treatment.

✓ Too low number of spermatozoa in the ejaculate for standard AI, IUI or IVF treatment.

Indications of ICSI with Epididymal Spermatozoa

✓ Epididymal spermatozoa can be obtained by microsurgical epididymal sperm aspiration (MESA) in the following conditions

- Congenital bilateral absence of the vas deferens
- Failed vasoepididymostomy
- Failed vasovasostomy
- Azoospermia because of bilateral hernia
- Obstructions at the level of both ejaculatory ducts
- Anejaculation because of spinal cord injury
- Retrograde ejaculation
- Other sexual dysfunction

Indications for ICSI with Testicular Spermatozoa

- All indications for MESA (above)
- Extensive scarring rendering MESA impossible
- Germ-cell hypoplasia: hypospermatogenesis
- Germ-cell aplasia with focal spermatogenesis
- Sertoli cell-only syndrome with focal spermatogenesis

Results

✓ The results of ICSI with ejaculated, epididymal, and testicular spermatozoa in terms of fertilization, embryo cleavage, and implantation rate after transfer can be considered to be similar to the results of standard IVF treatment in infertile couples with non-andrological infertility (Table 12-3).

✓ In the horse, ICSI has resulted in several foals being born worldwide. The inability of in vitro culture techniques to support equine embryo development once fertilization and initial cleavage divisions have occurred, requires oviductal transfer into recipient mares for success (see Zygote Intrafallopian Transfer, ZIFT).

⦿ See CD for demonstration of the ICSI procedure (Video 12-1).

Table 12-3
Summary of the Results of Four Years of ICSI (1991-1994) as Collected by the European Society for Human Reproduction and Endocrinology (ESHRE) Task Force on ICSI. The results of the first survey with the date until December 31, 1993 were published in Human Reproduction Update.

Parameter	Ejaculated	Epididymal	Testicular
Number of cycles	13,178	539	193
Oocytes injected	111,291	5744	2057
% intact after ICSI	90.3	91.9	89.6
% of intact oocytes	58.5	50.4	50 9
% transferred embryos	69.2	61.4	71.9
% embryo transfers	91.1	93.3	87.6
% positive HCG/cycle	28.7	34.9	33.2

Intrafollicular Insemination (IFI)

Background

✓ Intrafollicular insemination is an ART that has produced offspring in humans.

Indications

✓ The primary reasons are to circumvent the hostile uterine environment and to avoid post-mating induced endometritis. It may also have a place in stallions with few sperm numbers per ejaculate, or in conservation of cryopreserved stallion sperm resources.

✓ IFI has been attempted in horses, but to date no foals have been successfully produced from this technique.

In Vitro Fertilization (IVF)

Background

✓ The technique of in vitro fertilization (IVF) attempts to bring about the fusion of egg and the sperm in the laboratory instead of in the female's Fallopian tube (oviduct). Thanks to this technique there are now tens of thousands of children who have been born throughout the world, but very few horses.

Procedure

✓ IVF technology involves superovulation (ovarian hyperstimulation) in order to obtain multiple oocytes, thus increasing the odds for more embryos, from which more pregnancies might be achieved. Oocytes obtained by follicular aspiration (see below) are matured and then incubated with appropriately prepared capacitated spermatozoa from the male. If fertilization occurs within 48 hours, the embryos are cultured and then transferred to the uterus between day 2 and day 6 after fertilization.

✓ The efficiency of human IVF is high and approximately one in every 4-5 women who undergo the attempt achieve pregnancy. IVF is the therapeutic option of reproductive medicine with the highest yield per attempt, close on many occasions to that achieved by fertile couples with natural conception.

Indications

✓ The original indication for IVF was irreversible pathology of the Fallopian tubes, resulting from an inflammatory process (pelvic inflammatory disease) or previous surgery. In recent years, the indication for IVF when an abnormal male factor is present has become more common. There are other indications such as unexplained infertility, residual endometriosis, and infertility of immunological origin, which can also benefit from the application of IVF.

Techniques Derived from IVF

For patients with undamaged uterine tubes there has been increasing use of GIFT, zygote transfer (ZIFT) or of tubal embryo transfer (TET). GIFT is associated with higher levels of pregnancy than IVF but it has the drawback that it is unable to demonstrate the fertilizing capacity of the gametes. As far as ZIFT and TET technologies are concerned, they are usually applied in cases of infertility due to a male factor, an immunological factor, or unknown cause, provided that at least one donor uterine tube is normal.

✓ IVF in the horse is not repeatably successful. Only 2 foals have reportedly been born from IVF, both from oocytes matured in vivo. The primary barrier(s) to fertilization in equine IVF systems is zona penetration (± sperm capacitation).

✓ Various techniques have been published which are reported to have had some success.

From 159 oocytes that were collected non-surgically:

41 were fertilized by stallion semen treated with a calcium-ionophore

16 of these cleaved

8 were transferred into the ampullae of recipient mares

and 1 pregnancy resulted, this mare foaled.

Oocyte Retrieval / Ovum Pick-up / Follicular Aspiration

Percutaneous Through the Flank Technique

✓ Up to 60-70% successful, using a double lumen, 12-13 gauge needle providing the ability for continuous irrigation – aspiration of follicular contents.

Transvaginal Ultrasound-guided Technique

✓ Up to 40-60% successful, the best results were associated with use of an 18-gauge double lumen needle using continuous irrigation-aspiration; others have used a single lumen 12- or 16-gauge needle with an alternating push-pull technique to irrigate and aspirate follicular contents.

✓ Immature follicle aspiration is less rewarding than mature follicle aspiration. The greatest success is with aspiration of the dominant follicle 30-36 hours after stimulation with hCG. Use of a GnRH-analogue (deslorelin) as the means of stimulating follicle development and in vivo oocyte maturation has produced comparable results.

✓ Oocytes collected 20-24 hours after hCG administration (to promote in vivo maturation) should be cultured for 12-16 hours before transfer, or placed into the oviducts of recipient mare(s) who have been bred 12-24 hours prior to the transfer with semen from a highly fertile stallion.

✓ A typical oocyte culture system for in vitro maturation, IVM, would include a basic medium such as TCM-199, with 10% fetal calf serum, antibiotics as above for embryo transfer media, and pyruvate. The culture system should be at 38-39°C in an environment of 5%-6% CO_2 and air.

✓ Transvaginal ultrasound-guided technique to collect multiple follicles from the same mare can be accomplished. The mare's dominant follicle is aspirated first, then the remainder of her follicles that develop further on both ovaries are aspirated 3 days later. This was reported to have a 60% success rate.

✓ Transvaginal ultrasound-guided technique to collect multiple follicles from pregnant mares has also been reported. Oocyte collection was performed between days 20 to 150 of gestation. This resulted in a retrieval success of 152 oocytes from 304 follicles from 10 pregnant mares (50% success). The mean number of oocytes collected per mare was 2.7 per follicle aspiration attempt.

Oocyte Transfer or Intrafollicular Transfer of Oocytes (IFTO)

✓ Circumvents the problems of in vitro maturation (IVM) of oocytes, IVF, and ZIFT, or ET.

✓ Requires a normal recipient mare. The oocyte(s) can be transferred into her oviduct or directly into one of her dominant follicles (IFTO).

✓ For oviductal transfer, a standing flank laparotomy is performed exposing the ovary and oviduct. The recipient mare's dominant follicle is aspirated and positive identification of her oocyte is made. The donor oocyte is placed in DPBS and aspirated into a fire-polished glass pipette for transfer. The oocyte deposition is made 3 cm into the infundibulum of the recipient mare. The recipient mare is inseminated by routine AI 12-24 hours prior to the oviductal transfer

✓ Recipient mares that are ovariectomized or in diestrus can be used for oviductal transfer. They are prepared with 3 mg estradiol for 3-6 days prior to transfer, and given 150-200 mg P4 after the transfer.

✓ Pregnancy rates from oocyte transfer have reportedly ranged from 35-80%. The success rate is highly dependent upon donor mare age, semen quality, and the training and expertise of the personnel performing the procedures.

Oocyte Cryopreservation

Introduction

✓ The first birth following cryopreservation of human oocytes was in 1986, but there have been few births reported since. The intention with oocyte cryopreservation would be to freeze, thaw, and then fertilize by GIFT, IVF, or ICSI at a later date.

Indications and Advantages

✓ To preserve fertility if ovarian function is about to be lost, such as from a side effect of treatment for a life-threatening disease in young women (or children). Typically this would involve cytotoxic drug therapy, radiotherapy or surgical removal of the ovary for malignancy. If surgery is urgent, eggs can be retrieved from unstimulated ovaries.

Problems and Reservations

✓ There remain significant technical problems with the use of cryopreserved oocytes in ART. With current techniques it appears that mature eggs frozen, thawed and fertilized by IVF or ICSI have about half the pregnancy potential of eggs fertilized and frozen as embryos. There are still some concerns that fully mature (metaphase II) eggs are at a delicate stage where they may be vulnerable to chromosomal damage by freezing. On the other hand, immature eggs are more robust but generally cannot be matured to metaphase II after thawing.

Recommendations

Oocyte freezing is recommended for young females who are about to loose ovarian function. Oocyte freezing is not reliable enough to recommend for preservation of excess eggs in routine IVF or GIFT. This may become a potential ART useful in performance mares, harvesting and preserving her "young" more viable oocytes early in life for use later after she proves her value in the show ring or following a successful racing career.

✓ In 2001, the first foals were born from cryopreserved oocytes. The technique used was a vitrification process. Vitrification involves the use of very high concentrations of cryoprotectant to permeate the oocyte quickly inducing high viscosity of the fluid portions of the ooplasma, minimizing damaging ice crystal formation.

✓ Oocyte transfer into the oviducts of normal recipient mares was performed with 26 thawed oocytes, that were cultured for 12 hours after thawing. Three embryos developed and two foals were delivered from two mares.

Xenogeneic Gamete Intrafallopian Transfer (X-GIFT)

✓ Indications are as above for GIFT.

✓ One report involved 15 mare oocytes transferred into rabbit oviducts, 100,000 stallion sperm (raw) were placed into the same oviducts which were ligated to prevent loss of the gametes. Eight unfertilized oocytes were recovered. Failure of this procedure was thought to have been related due to a lack of adequate sperm preparation (capacitation?).

Zygote Intrafallopian Transfer Procedure (ZIFT)

✓ An ART in which ova are removed from a donor female by various methods, and undergo IVF with a donor male's spermatozoa. The resulting zygote(s) are transferred into the uterine tubes of the recipient female via laparoscopy or laparotomy. Embryo transfer (ET) is the predecessor to this technique (Figure 12-6). ⊙

✓ ZIFT is presently used in equine ART following ICSI fertilization procedures due to the present inefficiency of *in vitro* culture methods to support equine embryo growth and development to the blastocyst stage, where routine ET (intrauterine transfer) could then be performed.

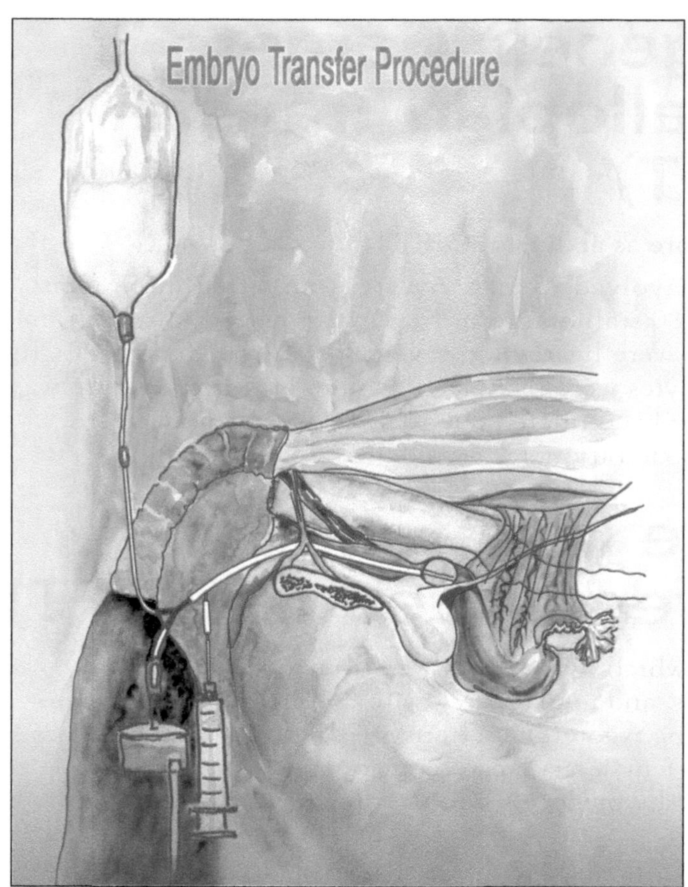

Figure 12-6 Illustration of the embryo flush procedure in the mare.

Glossary of Reproductive Terms

AI: Artificial insemination.

Anechoic: A term used in describing structures observed by ultrasonography referring to lack or absence of echo (sound wave) return, such as is seen with water.

Anestrus: The physiological period or abnormal condition in which there is an absence of estrous cycle activity and behavior due to pathological or seasonal influences.

Aneuploidy: Any deviation from an exact multiple of the haploid chromosome number.

ART: Assisted reproductive technology.

Atony: Lack of physiological tone especially of a contractile organ.

Barren: A mare that has failed to conceive in the most recent breeding season, or one more distant and not since. She may have conceived, been confirmed as pregnant, and then subsequently aborted, or had a stillbirth, and fit into the barren category.

Bicornual: Referring to both uterine horns.

Broad ligament: Suspends the uterine body and horns to the abdominal and pelvic walls. It originates in the lateral sublumbar region (from the 3rd or 4th lumbar to the 4th sacral vertebra), and the lateral pelvic walls, and extends to the dorsal, or attached border of the uterine horns and the lateral margins of the uterine body. (aka: mesometrium).

Capacitation: The change that sperm undergo in the female reproductive tract that enables them to acrosome react and penetrate and fertilize an egg.

Caslick surgery (Caslick's): See vulvoplasty.

Cervix: Is the constricted, thick-walled, muscular extension of the uterine body that is 5.0 to 7.5 cm in length. Its distal end projects caudally into the anterior vagina and is referred to as the external os cervix.

Chimerism: The presence of two cell lines within an individual that are of different origin as from a twin.

Circadian (q24h): Occurring every 24 hours, or daily.

Circalunar (q29d): Occurring once a month or lunar cycle.

Circannual (q1y): Occurring once per annum or yearly.

Clitoris: The female homologue of the penis.

Cloning: The process of producing an individual grown from a single somatic cell of its parent that is genetically identical to it.

Conception Rate (CR): Is defined as the number of mares that are diagnosed pregnant between 9-17 days post-ovulation compared with the total number of mares bred.

Corpus Hemorrhagicum (CH): The structure that fills with blood following ovulation of the mature or Graafian follicle. The fibrin within serves as the lattice-work for invasion of the luteal cells which fill its cavity to form the corpus luteum (CL), usually by Day 5-6 in the mare.

Corpus Luteum (CL): The structure that develops from the CH above, is filled with luteal cells and secretes progesterone (P4). Its typical lifespan in the mare is around 85 days, if not caused to regress by endogenous or exogenous prostaglandin F2-a (PGF2). [Plural: corpora lutea; CLs]

Cytokine: Any of a class of immunoregulatory substances (as lymphokines) that are secreted by cells of the immune system.

Deslorelin (Ovuplant™): A GnRH analog.

Diestrus: The physiological period or condition dominated by a corpus luteum (CL) under the primary influence of progesterone and behaviorally not receptive to breeding. (aka: cold, out, not showing, not in or not in heat)

Diurnal: Occurring during the day.

Early Embryonic Death (EED): Is defined as the loss of the conceptus or embryo between days 9 to 45; usually after day 18 and before day 36.

Ecbolic: A drug (ergot alkaloids, oxytocin, or PGF) that tends to increase uterine contractions and were designed originally to facilitate parturition.

eCG: Equine chorionic gonadotropin or pregnant mare serum gonadotropin (PMSG); can be used as a hormonal (blood) test indicative of pregnancy.

Efficiency: The quality or degree of being efficient, which means productive of the desired effect, especially productive without waste.

Endometrial Angiosis: A degenerative process affecting uterine vasculature that is a result of aging and is aggravated by multiple pregnancies.

Endometritis: An acute or chronic-active inflammation of the endometrium and its associated cellular components and structures.Typically in the mare, the inflammation does not extend deeper than the endometrial layer, sparing the myometrial and serosal layers. More extensive inflammation of uterine tissues (i.e., metritis or perimetritis) may be encountered in postpartum mares.

Endometriosis: The presence and growth of functional endometrial tissue in places other than the uterus that often results in severe pain and infertility.

Endometrosis: This is a term used to describe the wide range of degenerative histopathologic characteristics of the endometrium of mares. This condition is degenerative (but not necessarily age-related) and lacks the typical features of active inflammation. Infiltrates of lymphocytes, plasmacytes and macrophages are the predominating cell types observed in biopsy samples of the endometrium. There are various degrees of fibrosis in and around endometrial glandular structures, lymphatic vessel dilatation and areas of stasis, and endometrial glandular and lymphatic cysts. A development of 'wear and tear' during the reproductively active life of the mare.

Endometrium: The epithelial layer of the uterus which is a simple layer of columnar, cuboidal to tall epithelial cells, dependent upon the stage of the estrous cycle. Branching tubular endometrial glands extend from their openings at the epithelial surface through the compact layer of the lamina propria to the spongy layer located just beneath the inner circular layer of smooth muscle of the myometrium

Estradiol (E2): Estrogen is the key hormone promoting folliculogenesis and for triggering the physiologic events necessary for receptive reproductive behavior. The dominant follicle(s) possess an enhanced capacity for estradiol synthesis and secretion over other follicles. Such a capacity involves the action of both follicle stimulating hormone (FSH) and luteinizing hormone (LH) on follicular theca and granulosa cells. Estradiol is a phenolic steroid alcohol C18H24O2

Estrous Cycle: The events typically defined as beginning with an ovulation (Day 0) and ending the day before the next ovulation and includes the physiologic and behavioral events of estrus and diestrus. The average inter-ovulatory interval for most mares is 21 days, but the range can be from 18 to 24 days. The estrous phase (follicular phase) may last from 3 to 7 days, and is dominated by one or more large (> 30 mm dia.), pre-ovulatory (aka, Graafian) follicles, estrogen17β (E2), and behavioral signs of heat, or receptivity to the stallion. The diestrous phase (luteal phase) lasts 13 to 17 days, and is dominated by a corpus luteum (CL; or more than one corpora lutea, CLs), progesterone (P4), and behavioral signs indicating non-receptivity to the approach of the stallion.

Estrus: The physiological period or condition dominated by a large follicle (or more than one follicle) that is approaching ovulation and under the primary influence of estrogen; behaviorally the female is receptive to breeding (aka: in heat, teasing in, hot, or showing).

ET: Embryo transfer (NOT the movie).

Graafian follicle: a mature follicle in a mammalian ovary that contains a liquid-filled cavity and that ruptures during ovulation to release an egg.

Fallopian Tube(s): See Oviduct.

Fertility: The quality or state of being fertile, which means producing or being capable of producing offspring; it implies the power or ability to reproduce in kind or to assist in reproduction and growth.

Fimbrial Cysts (hydatids of Morgagni): Are common in mares. They frequently are pedunculated, and histologically are lined with ciliated columnar epithelium, indicating that they are of Mullerian duct origin.

Flagging: Rhythmic up and down motion of the stallion's tail that usually accompanies ejaculation.

Flehmen: A response by the stallion or mare (i.e., upper lip curl) that is an indication that either has detected a pleasing odor or pheromone.

Folliculogenesis: Is a physiologic process that can be divided into three phases: recruitment, selection, and dominance. Follicles undergo atresia (apoptoisis or degeneration), ovulation, or spontaneous luteinization.

Fossal Cysts: May be found in the region of the ovulation fossa.

These are similar to fimbrial cysts, and their impact on fertility of the mare is open to question.

FSH: Follicle stimulating hormone; a hormone from an anterior lobe of the pituitary gland that stimulates the growth of follicles in the ovary.

GIFT: Gamete intrafallopian transfer

Gonadotropin (gonoadotrophin): Human chorionic gonadotropin (hCG) and gonadotropin-releasing hormone (GnRH).

GnRH: Gonadotropin releasing hormone; a decapeptide hormone produced by the hypothalamus that stimulates the adenohypophysis to release luteinizing hormone and follicle-stimulating hormone.

hCG: Human chorionic gonadotropin; a product of placental origin that is isolated and purified from the urine of pregnant women; its effect in the mare (and other species) is similar to luteinizing hormone (LH).

Hermaphrodite: Anomalous differentiation of the gonads with both ovarian and testicular tissues present.

Hinny: The resultant offspring between a mating of a jack (male donkey) and a mare (female horse).

Hydrometra: Accumulation of serous or watery secretions in the uterine cavity, as opposed to mucous or purulent material.

Hyperechoic: Increased tissue density as indicated by a higher rate of echo or sound wave return compared with surrounding structures.

Hypoechoic: Decreased tissue density as indicated by a lower rate of echo or sound wave return compared with surrounding structures.

Hypoplasia: Under-developed, smaller than normal development.

Hysterectomy: Surgical removal of the uterus.

Hysteroscopy: A procedure in which direct visualization of the uterine cavity (lumen) is accomplished using a fiberoptic endoscope or similar instrument.

ICSI: Intracytoplasmic sperm injection.

Infertility: The condition of being not fertile or barren.

Infundibulum: Funnel-shaped portion of the oviduct.

Inhibin: Glycoprotein hormone that acts upon the pituitary gland; in the male it is secreted by the Sertoli cells of the testicle; in the female it is secreted by the granulosa cells of the ovarian follicle; its function is to inhibit the secretion of follicle stimulating hormone (FSH).

In hand: Maintaining restraint and control of the stallion and/or mare using a halter and lead rope; usually refers to breeding by live cover or natural mating.

Intersex: See hermaphrodite, pseudohermaphrodite, and male pseudohermaphrodite.

Intromission: Penetration of the vagina by the erect penis.

IVF: In vitro fertilization.

IVM: In vitro maturation of oocyte(s).

Karyotype: The chromosomal characteristics of a cell, includes identification of the somatic chromosome number and the sex chromosomes.

Klinefelter's Syndrome: Male phenotype with excess of one sex chromosome (47XXY in the human, or Polysomy X)

Lactating: A mare that has "proven" herself reproductively, has a foal at her side, and is lactating; the result of having recently conceived, successfully gestated, and foaled. She may also be referred to as a 'wet', foaling or postpartum mare.

Laparoscopy: Visual examination of the inside of the abdomen using a laparoscope.

Laparotomy: Surgical invasion of the abdominal wall.

Lavage: Washing; the therapeutic washing out of an organ, area or body part.

LH: Luteinizing hormone; a hormone of protein-carbohydrate composition that is obtained from the adenohypophysis of the pituitary gland and that in the female stimulates ovulation, the development of the corpus luteum, and with follicle-stimulating hormone the secretion of progesterone.

Luteolysis: Lysis of the corpus luteum (CL).

Maiden: A mare that has never been bred or exposed to a stallion for breeding purposes. She would be considered nulliparous.

Male Pseudohermaphrodite: Testicular gonadal tissues but female secondary sex characteristics; karyotype = XX.

Melatonin: Secreted from the pineal during the night, is involved in the regulation of circadian rhythms. Melatonin effects the neural and metabolic activity of SCN neurons directly by high-affinity melatonin receptors located within SCN. Melatonin indirectly inhibits gonadal function through its target tissue in the SCN. Its effective action is antagonistic to GnRH production and release from the hypothalamus.

Metritis: Inflammation of the uterus, involving the endometrium and myometrium.

Mosaicism: The presence of two or more cell lines that are genotypically distinct within the same individual, derived from a single zygote.

Mucometra: Accumulation of mucous secretion in the uterine cavity, devoid of inflammatory cellular components.

Mule: The resultant offspring between the mating of a stallion (male horse) and a jenny (female donkey).

Multiparous: Having had multiple births.

Nocturnal: Occurring during the night.

Nuclear transfer (NT): The process in which the nucleus of a somatic cell is removed and placed into the cytoplasm of a recipient cell that has had its own nucleus removed; a process used in cloning.

Nulliparous: Having never given birth.

Nyctohemeral: Occurs during both night and day.

Oocyte: Ovum, egg. The female gamete that has a haploid number of chromosomes; equine oocytes, like those of other species, are ovulated as 2° oocytes, not as 1° oocytes

Oogenesis: Is the process of development of the ovum within the follicle. It begins with oogonia, which originate from primordial germ cells in the embryo.

Opsonin: An antibody of blood serum that makes foreign cells or antigens more susceptible to phagocytosis.

OT: Oocyte transfer

Oviduct: Salpinx, uterine tube, or Fallopian tube. Its three parts are the isthmus, the ampulla, and the infundibulum.

Ovarian bursa: Of the mare is a pouch lined by peritoneum. It extends from the ovulation fossa caudally to the cranial aspect of the uterine horn. Its lateral bounds are formed by the uterine tube and its mesosalpinx. Its medial bounds are formed by the proper ligament of the ovary, which is a fold of the broad ligament.

Ovariectomy: Surgical removal of the ovaries.

Oxytocin: A posterior pituitary octapeptide hormone C43H66N12O12S2 that stimulates the contraction of uterine muscle and the secretion of milk.

Paraovarian or Tubal Cysts: Are remnants of the mesonephric duct system. These may be found in the mesosalpinx or mesovarium and be from 2 to 50 mm in diameter.

Perineum: The body wall encompassing the outlet of the pelvis, and surrounding the urogenital tract outlet, and the distal rectum and anus.

PGF: Prostaglandin F; an oxygenated unsaturated cyclic fatty acid hormone having effects upon smooth muscle of the uterus, intestine, and blood vessels.

Phallectomy: Surgical removal or resection of the penis.

Pineal gland: Is an outgrowth of the forebrain. In man its functions are obscure, but in other vertebrates it acts as an endocrine gland, secreting the hormone melatonin. Melatonin: Is secreted primarily during the night (dark hours). Light stimulus via the RHT inhibits melatonin synthesis and release.

Pneumovagina: The abnormal condition in which the mare aspirates air into the vagina and potentially the cervix and uterus during respiration or physical exertion.

Polar Body: The discarded half-complement of chromosomes that is sequestered inside the mature oocyte.

Polyploidy: Having more than two full sets of homologous chromosomes

Pregnancy Rate (PR): The number of mares pregnant at day 45 (or beyond) compared with the total number of mares bred. This parameter may be calculated based on single estrous cycle, monthly or seasonal intervals.

Progesterone (P4): A steroid sex hormone C21H30O2 that is secreted by the corpus luteum to prepare the endometrium for embryo and fetal support and development and later during pregnancy is produced by the placenta.

Progestogen: Progestagen, progestin, progesterone, P4; any of several progestational steroids.

Pseudohermaphrodite: An individual exhibiting the condition of having the gonads of one sex and the external genitalia and other sex organs so variably developed that the apparent sex of the individual is uncertain.

Pyometra: Accumulation of purulent (inflammatory) secretion in the uterine cavity.

PZD: Partial zona dissection, as associated with IVF.

Quotidian: Occurring every day

Relaxin: A protein hormone that is thought to act synergistically with progesterone to maintain pregnancy and to promote loosening of pelvic ligaments at the time of parturition; a polypeptide sex hormone of the corpus luteum.

Reproductive Efficiency: The ability to produce offspring in a positive and effective manner without waste.

Retinohypothalamic Tract (RHT or RHP): The pathway from the retina to the SCN. Prominent regulators include glutamate, acetylcholine and melatonin.

Seasonally Polyestrous: There is a defined period of time during the year in which the female exhibits cyclical or repetitive signs of estrus in response to her reproductive physiology as determined by follicle development, production of estrogen, ovulation, CL development, production of progesterone, and if she does not conceive, repetition of the same events (usually) on a regular or somewhat predictable interval.

Salpingitis: Inflammation of the uterine tube or oviduct (salpinx).

Serviceable: The most useful term, as it implies the relationship of physical capability to intended use.

Soundness: Implies an absolute understanding, which when used for the purpose of a mare's breeding soundness examination is potentially misleading.

Sterile: Failing to produce or incapable of producing offspring

Subfertility: The condition of being less than normally fertile though still capable of effecting fertilization; reduced reproductive efficiency.

Suitable: A term of art and refers to temperament, ability, and relationship of the horse to rider, driver, exhibitor, or other desired use.

Superovulation: In the human this is referred to as controlled ovarian hyperstimulation, in animals the technique involves administration of gonadotropins to stimulate folliculogenesis toward development of multiple dominant follicles.

Suprachiasmatic Nucleus (SCN): Of the hypothalamus sustains a stable circadian rhythm of neuronal activity. The phase of this rhythm can be reset by neural signals from other brain sites in a time-of-day dependent manner.

SUZI: Subzonal insemination of sperm; stops short of penetrating the oocyte plasma membrane in contrast to ICSI in which one sperm is deposited directly in the ooplasma.

TET: Tubal embryo transfer.

Trisomy: The presence of an additional (3rd) chromosome of one type (2n + 1) in an otherwise diploid genotype (autosomal; e.g. Down's Syndrome, trisomy 21)

Turner's Syndrome: Female phenotype with lack of one sex chromosome (45XO or 45X in the human, or Monosomy X)

Unicornual: Referring to one of the uterine horns, but not both.

Urometra: Accumulation of urine in the uterine cavity.

Uterotubal Junction (UTJ): The junction between the distal isthmus of the oviduct (uterine tube) and the tip of the uterine horn. In the mare, this is a distinct papilla surrounded by circular smooth muscle fibers forming a sphincter.

Vagina: Joins the vestibule with the cervix. It ends caudally at the transverse fold above the external urethral opening where it is contiguous with the vestibule. The transverse fold is a remnant of the hymen, which partitioned the vestibule from the vagina proper during embryogenesis. The transverse fold marks the line of merger between the cranial portion of the reproductive tract, which is of mesodermal origin, and the caudal portion, which, as stated above, is of ectodermal origin. The vagina may be up to 20 cm in depth. The vaginal fornix is an annular recess formed by the joining of the cranial vaginal walls and the vaginal portion (external os) of the uterine cervix.

Vaginoscopy: Direct visualization of the anterior vaginal cavity, fornix, and external os cervix using a sterile, stainless steel Thoroughbred or disposable cardboard or plastic speculum.

Vernal: Of, relating to, or occurring in the spring

Vestibule: The tubular portion of the vulva connecting the labia with the vagina.

Vitrification: A method of cellular cryopreservation. Vitrification involves the use of very high concentrations of a cryoprotectant to permeate the oocyte or embryo very quickly to induce a high viscosity of the fluid portions of the ooplasma or trophoblast and minimize damaging ice crystal formation.

Vulva: That portion of the genital tract common to both the urinary and reproductive systems. It includes two labia, and the clitoris with its associated sinuses, fossa and glans.

Vulvoplasty: Corrective surgery to reduce the effective length (opening) of the lips of the vulva to prevent pneumovagina.

Wet Mare: See Lactating.

Wind-sucking: See pneumovagina.

ZIFT: Zygote intrafallopian transfer.

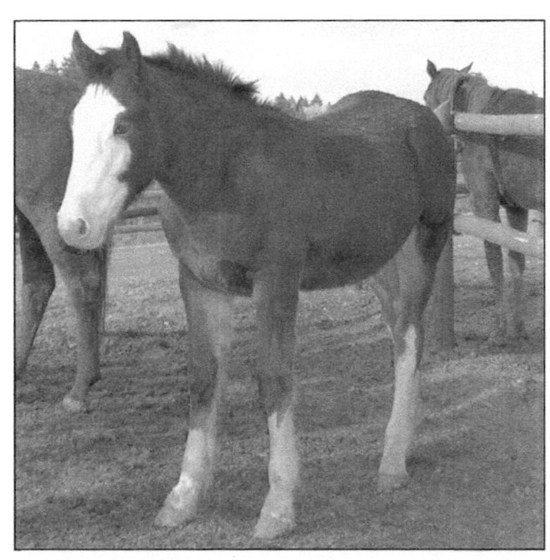

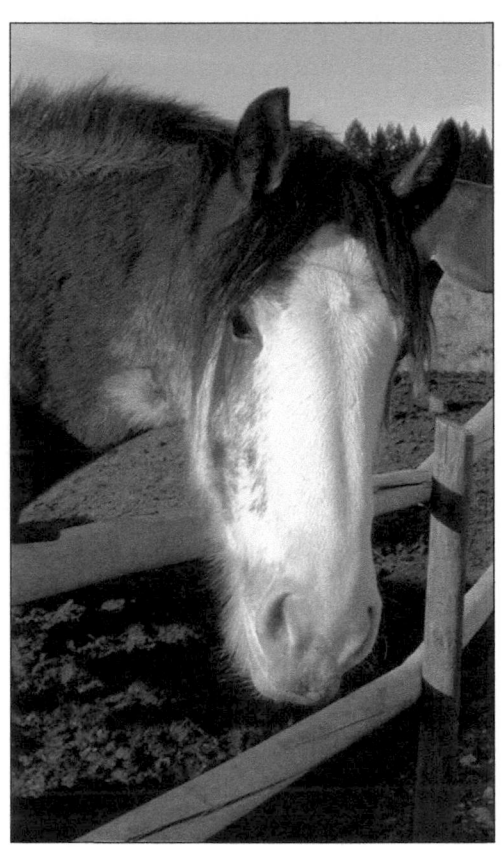

Index

Page numbers followed by an *f* indicate a figure; page numbers followed by a *t* indicate a table.

C

D

E

F

G

H

I

J

N

O

P

Q

R

S

W

X

Y

Z

NOTES

NOTES

NOTES

We hope you enjoy this
Made Easy Series volume for the
Equine Practitioner.
If you would like more information on
other **Made Easy** Series
products please call 877-306-9793
or visit our online store at
www.veterinarywire.com

Available Titles in this Series-
for the Equine Practitioner
– Ophthalmology

Forthcoming Titles in this Series-
for the Equine Practitioner
– Wound Care
– Dermatology

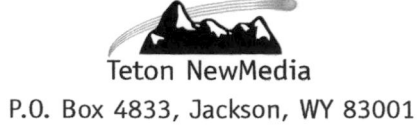

Teton NewMedia
P.O. Box 4833, Jackson, WY 83001

9781591610113